# PERFECT PRACTICE

*HOW TO BUILD A SUCCESSFUL FUNCTIONAL MEDICINE BUSINESS, ATTRACT YOUR IDEAL PATIENTS, SERVE YOUR COMMUNITY, AND GET PAID WHAT YOU'RE WORTH*

## BY SACHIN PATEL

---

### FREE PRACTICE RESOURCES

This book includes a series of additional tools, videos, and strategies that you can instantly implement into your practice in as little as three days!

Download your FREE resources here:
www.perfectpracticebook.com

---

**Legal and copyright**

Sachin Patel, DC
Living Proof Institute Inc.
77 City Centre Drive, Suite 501
Mississauga, ON, L5B 1M5
Canada
www.becomeproof.com

**Ordering information**

Quantity sales. Special discounts are available on quantity purchases by corporations, associations, and others. For details, contact the publisher at the address above.

First edition

Manufactured in Canada

## Introduction

Welcome healthcare hero!

I'm so grateful that I get to share this book with you. In these pages, you will discover dozens of ideas that can transform your life, practice, and community for the better.

As I am sure you've discovered, functional and lifestyle medicine can have a profound impact on one's health and vitality. In fact, I can almost guarantee that it has transformed your life or that of someone close to you.

Equipped with the knowledge to spare human suffering, many practitioners struggle to create the practice of their dreams. Not because they are incapable, but because we haven't made enough mistakes yet!

I wrote this book as part of my mission to accelerate the much-needed expansion of functional and lifestyle medicine into mainstream healthcare.

The intention of this book is to plant dozens of seeds in your mental garden, so that you can live a life of purpose and impact while working towards economic and geographic freedom.

In this book, you will learn how to attract the right patients, transform their lives, and make a living!

# Table of Contents

# ACKNOWLEDGMENTS

## DEDICATIONS AND THANK YOUS

This book is dedicated to my fellow heart-centered functional medicine practitioners, who are out there trying to make the world a better place for generations to come.

I would like to thank my wife, son, and parents for their endless support and for making all of my dreams comes true. I love you all dearly.

I'd also like to thank my brother, Ritesh Patel, for his continued inspiration to make me a better father, clinician, and entrepreneur.

Finally, a heartfelt thank you to my awesome team at the Living Proof Institute for their outstanding efforts and dedication to our patients and practitioners. I appreciate your trust as we navigate uncharted waters. The best is yet to come!

# ENDORSEMENTS FOR SACHIN PATEL

Shelly Sethi where to begin...? This mentorship has been the best decision for me with regards to where I spend my time, money and mental energy. I have explored and purchased other mentorship programs in the past couple of years, and found this one at exactly the right time, offering exactly what I need. The components I was missing in my business/practice development were efficient plans for marketing, practice model setup and most importantly personal mindset. The support of this community has been invaluable and I have changed my entire paradigm of who I am and what I can offer and how. I can't thank you enough!

Sara DeFrancesco The Living Proof Mentorship will change your mind, change your business, and change your life. The program, marketing, and public service taught in this program is the most cutting edge and the most heart and service centered in Functional Medicine. Sachin has taken his strengths in personal development, clinical skills, and next level entrepreneurship and combined them into a mentorship that is transformational. Stop wandering around in the dark and #becomeproof now.

Robert Inesta The Living Proof mentorship program is a must for functional medicine practitioners who want to make a massive impact and change the world. The team is amazing - cutting-edge clinicians, top-notch life and business coaching and an over abundance of life changing information that can be put into action immediately. All bases are covered. They consistently over-deliver and are always there to support you. I am truly grateful and honored to be a part of this program!

Buddy Touchinsky Hell, just being in this FB group alone is worth the price of admission. Imagine when we all have 2-3 years of experience under our belts. And I still can't wait for the LPI practitioner retreat where we rent a beach front in Costa Rica and we spend a week or two of intensive learning from each other and whomever else we fly in to teach us 😊

Josiah Smith Didn't think twice, never looked back. If you are seeking a turnkey functional medicine model in becoming the goto practitioner in your community that has a massive impact both in attracting and serving patients and your bottom line, look no further. Dr. Patel and his team over deliver and set you up for success.

## PERFECT PRACTICE CHECKLIST

The following checklist is a great way to evaluate your practice and your journey as a practitioner. Remember that this is a lifelong journey in both self-discovery and self-development. Every blank checkbox should be viewed as a growth opportunity, both personally and professionally.

Each topic is covered in this book, but you will find more in-depth information contained in our bonus materials and in our Facebook community page.

Go to www.perfectpracticebook.com for your bonus content and invitation to our private Facebook group.

## Personal development

- ❏ I practice what I preach to my patients
- ❏ I have time for myself to pursue personal passion projects
- ❏ I have a heightened awareness of the words I use
- ❏ I have complete control of my thoughts
- ❏ I have an abundance mindset
- ❏ I am selective with my patients
- ❏ My DISC score is _____
- ❏ My KOLBE-A score is _____
- ❏ My love language is _____
- ❏ My chronotype is _____
- ❏ I practice feng shui
- ❏ I run blood work and functional lab testing on myself
- ❏ I have an unfair advantage
- ❏ I have a mentor or coach to guide me personally and professionally

## Practice principles

- ❏ I have a smart overhead strategy
- ❏ I reinvest money back into my business, not just time
- ❏ I have explainer videos, so I don't have to repeat myself
- ❏ I use tools like Boomerang to ensure follow-up
- ❏ I provide automated education
- ❏ I have a signature gift for my patients to show gratitude
- ❏ I have personalized touch points
- ❏ I have automated touch points
- ❏ I create a unique user experience
- ❏ I have a follow-up strategy with patients
- ❏ I have great experiential strategies
- ❏ I have an amazing team that support "our" mission
- ❏ I use personality testing to learn more about myself and my team

## Digital tools

- ❏ I have an autoresponder and CRM software (Active Campaign http://bit.ly/lpiactivecampaign)
- ❏ I have a lead capture software (Click Funnels http://bit.ly/lpiclick)
- ❏ I have a webinar software (Zoom http://bit.ly/lpizoom)
- ❏ I have an awesome mobile-friendly website that captures leads
- ❏ I have a SNAP download
- ❏ I have a quiz on my website to survey and qualify leads

## Money mindset

- ❏ I contribute to a cause greater than myself and my practice
- ❏ I have karmic currency
- ❏ My clients see great value in my services

## Marketing and messaging

- ❑ I am a polished public speaker
- ❑ I deliver free workshops or webinars at least once a month
- ❑ I have defined my *hero's journey* and feel comfortable sharing it
- ❑ I have a scalable marketing formula that works
- ❑ I measure my marketing outcomes
- ❑ I ask for the sale, but not too often
- ❑ I explain things in a very simple way (fifth-grade level)
- ❑ I am consistent in my efforts
- ❑ I have identified my avatar
- ❑ I am the avatar my patients are looking for
- ❑ I have a niche audience that I market to
- ❑ I have a signature opt-in (www.30in30.org)
- ❑ I have a signature talk ("Doctor of the Future")
- ❑ I have a signature program (www.lpiessentials.com)
- ❑ I use analogies to explain things
- ❑ I have created a "Consumer's Guide"
- ❑ I survey my audience before I create products or content
- ❑ I create content that can be repurposed
- ❑ I use the star, story, solution method
- ❑ I have a character diamond
- ❑ I convert prospects into patients through tension, not pressure
- ❑ I have a post-workshop follow-up sequence to build authority
- ❑ I am actively asking for referrals
- ❑ I leverage automation
- ❑ I share my successes
- ❑ I regularly collect testimonials from patients

## Facebook Strategy

- ❑ I have a social media strategy
- ❑ I have a business page for my practice
- ❑ I have a group that I manage
- ❑ I fully express my values and polarize my audience
- ❑ I keep my content relevant
- ❑ I spend money on Facebook ads
- ❑ I look at my analytics
- ❑ I engage with my posts in a strategic way
- ❑ I create video content on Facebook
- ❑ I repurpose my video content
- ❑ I do Facebook LIVE events and have a strategy
- ❑ I use retargeting pixels

## MY JOURNEY . . .

In November 2004, I graduated from New York Chiropractic School as one of the top students in my class, and I landed my dream job in Cincinnati, Ohio. I was working with elite athletes, marathon runners, and even Olympic gold medalists. I loved it; life was really great!

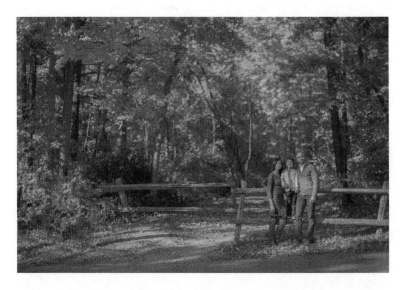

I spent two years working hard at growing my associateship. I have a reliable work ethic, so the practice grew organically over time.

Then in the fall of 2006, my life completely changed. Our practice was asked to be on the evening news for a feature story. One of our patients loved our services so much she wanted to help spread the message.

My boss at the time had frozen on live television before this and declined the interview. Instead, she asked me to do it. I was nervous at first, but then I became excited because this was my chance.

Two years into practice, I loved what I was doing. I was working with some amazing people. This was my chance to make a huge impact in my community.

The news story was all about tennis elbow and golfer's elbow. Our practice was using a revolutionary soft tissue therapy called Active Release Technique that was producing remarkable results.

The filming was done in August, and the story aired in October. It aired at 5:20 pm. I remember this because, at 5:21 pm, our phone was ringing off the hook. Of course, I got excited because I loved my job! I love helping people, and I love making a difference in people's lives.

**The moment of truth**

As a result of this news report, my life path was altered in a way I had never imagined. As these new patients started coming in, our office demographic changed overnight. We went from seeing some of the healthiest people in our community to seeing some of the sickest.

For a chiropractor working in a sports office, this was a very foreign sight to me. As I started taking histories on these patients, I instantly realized that there was not much I could do for them. They were dealing with autoimmunity, chronic fatigue, fibromyalgia, and other chronic illnesses.

My training and my work over the prior two years had not prepared me for this moment in time. After going through patients' histories, I realized that there was nowhere else I could even refer them to because they had already been to "every" specialist and had "every" scan.

My wife, who is a pharmacist, could not help me because these people had already exhausted every single drug for their diagnosis.

Since I didn't know where to send them, at that moment, I had a very clear revelation that I needed to become the person to help them and many others (as I discovered) who were looking for answers.

I didn't even know where to start. By coincidence, I started getting case studies emailed to me from a fellow chiropractor (Dr. Ron

Grisanti), that resembled my struggling patients. I started reviewing these case studies and it all made perfect sense. Fix the root cause!

I started diving deeper into the case studies, and this is how I discovered functional medicine. I had no idea that addressing these complex issues with root cause resolution was actually within my scope of practice, a whole new world opened up for me!

Through all of this, I realized I had the potential to help patients finally find some answers to their chronic health issues.

When Dr. Grisanti offered his training program, I was one of the first students to enroll. I was proudly part of the first graduating class of Functional Medicine University.

To be honest, I took that course reluctantly because I already had my perfect job. However, I had a deep desire to find out if there was anything that could be done to help those people who were now turning to me for help.

I convinced myself that I would do the course for myself. I had my own health challenges at the time. I was experiencing digestive issues, persistent acne, and joint stiffness.

I took the course selfishly for myself, but what I learned made me realize that I could not go back to working in the same capacity as before. I could not go back to just helping people with their soft tissue and musculoskeletal problems.

I realized I had a whole new tool I could use to help these same people and get outstanding clinical outcomes for them.

Functional Medicine changed my life and my clinical perspective, but most importantly it enhanced my ability to serve my community.

My boss didn't understand it though, and she had already developed and created this amazing soft tissue practice. Changing and evolving her practice was not her top priority. I don't blame her.

## The test

When it came time for me to take over the practice, I had to kindly turn down the offer. It was a difficult thing to do, because I had worked so hard to help build that practice up. It was the right thing for me to do at the time.

My friend and colleague Dr. Fuad Amer and I decided to look into opening a practice together. We were soon presented with an opportunity to work for a company to help them develop their existing practices, located in high-traffic gyms.

Dr. Amer and I jumped at the opportunity and worked to quickly grow the practices. We started doing extremely well and were helping a lot of patients.

We offered chiropractic care, massage therapy, functional medicine, nutritional consulting, and more. We both fell in love with our careers again!

Things were going really well. Two years in, I've got my real dream job. I've got my dream home. My wife was able to stay at home (and quit her draining job as a pharmacist) after my son's birth. I was making enough money to support our family, and I was delivering my dream services to my dream patients.

## The price of success

With our rapid growth came rapid expansion and income. Our practices were so successful that the company started to aggressively expand across the East Coast of the US in hopes to replicate the same outcomes. We had helped them create a profitable business model.

As they started to expand, they made a few errors that would prove to be fatal to their business. Their poor judgment led to delayed payments, partial payments, and eventually IOUs. Despite the financial turbulence, I stayed on for another eight months in the hopes that things would turn around. Almost overnight my life flipped upside down.

I was in trouble. My wife was a year out of work, my son was a year old, and my parents had moved in with me. I had a new home I had just built, and the company I was working for owed me $60,000 that they could not afford to pay me.

I was loyal and committed to my patients, so I kept working for the company to fulfill my obligations. When they offered me shares in the organization, I knew I would never see that money.

I was dying on the inside. I had plenty of sleepless nights and a crippling level of uncertainty.

**The nail in the coffin**

Then, at a friend's wedding in Hawaii, I sat on the beach and spilled the beans to my friend Shawn Williams. He said four words that would forever change my life: "Dude, you gotta leave."

A week later I built up enough courage to leave my role. It was extremely difficult, but I had no choice at this point. Out of money, out of options, but not out of hope. I knew I had a valuable gift that is needed by millions of people.

After much contemplation, I decided I was going to start my own functional medicine consulting practice. I had to reinvent myself. I was starting from scratch, and I had to find a new way to practice functional medicine on a shoestring budget because of how stretched I was.

What I needed to do was figure out a strategic way to launch a functional medicine business, have a smart overhead, and grow the practice.

I committed 110 percent to my success, but I was strapped for cash. So I took out a home equity line of credit to take some of the financial pressure off. I took out enough money to keep me afloat for three months.

The loan enabled me to take money off my mind so I could focus on being of service and helping people. I wanted to operate from a place of abundance instead of a position of scarcity.

I started looking for office space in my area. Most spaces required significant work, planning, and investment. I didn't have the time or the money to wait around. I needed to start working ASAP.

In search of the perfect office, I connected with a friend, Emily Gilmartin. Emily introduced me to a whole new office concept called co-working. My mind was blown!

She showed me a beautiful office that was fully furnished, with shared staffing, and equipped with fantastic amenities. It was a co-working space shared by accountants, lawyers, and other professionals – but rarely healthcare practitioners!

What's unique about functional medicine is that we don't need fancy equipment, mega staff, or the constant use of the boardroom and kitchen. The rent was only $1,000 a month with 60-day terms. It was a no-brainer.

**A new model of healthcare delivery was born!**

I was able to use technology, social media, strategy, and the wisdom from many mentors to go from having to manually generate patients to being able to automatically generate patients.

As I started seeing patients, our practice became instantly profitable. My stress declined significantly, and I was able to pay off the loan in two months. Our company has made a profit every single month since its inception.

I figured out a proven model: a cash-based functional medicine clinic with virtually no overhead and no capital investment costs. This model works in any city, in any country.

Since starting the Living Proof Institute in 2011, our team has built two successful offices (in the US and Canada) and worked with thousands of patients.

In 2013 other practitioners started to take notice and began reaching out for help. I have since helped over 100 functional medicine practitioners rediscover their passion, help more people in their communities, and earn what their knowledge and impact are worth.

Since embarking on this journey, our team and its influence have grown tremendously. It was hard work but worth every drop of sweat.

According to James Maskell, of *The Evolution of Medicine*, The Living Proof Institute is regarded as one of the "most innovative functional medicine practices in the world." I am so proud of our team and community for supporting our vision.

It has been a marvelous honor to serve others and share this message with the world. On my journey, I've had the pleasure of being part of some really cool conferences, private meetings, and mastermind groups.

I've worked with almost a dozen mentors who specialize in marketing and functional medicine, I've read over 200 books, I've delivered over 250 LIVE presentations and webinars, and I've posted on Facebook over 3,000 times!

To share my experiences, I've written this book to teach you the most important lessons I have learned. I want you to learn from my mistakes, so you don't waste any time. Your patients need you now more than ever.

There is nothing noble about reinventing the wheel, so let me walk you through the fundamental principles to help you attract your perfect patients, serve your community, and get paid what you're worth.

# WHY?

## Why Functional Medicine, Why Now?

Chances are if you're reading this book you're fully aware of the broken healthcare system we have. People are sicker than ever, taking more drugs than ever, at a higher cost than ever.

The ship is going to hit the iceberg; it's just a matter of when. There's also another important matter of who can help get as many people off the boat before it hits as possible and who is going to be there to save those drowning in the water?

Will it be you or the person down the street?

Let me let you in on a secret you might not know; it's going to take both of you!

There are so many chronically ill people right now that need your help. In fact, there is a huge shortage of trained and ready functional medicine practitioners.

We are the only ones that can save thousands of lives and prevent millions from suffering – but we ourselves are not ready for the tidal wave that's coming.

I wrote this book so that you can accelerate your role in your community as a healthcare hero. I'm going to share with you some of the most effective tools I've used to grow my practice and impact, while increasing my personal freedom.

There is a critical intersection taking place right now between the humanities and technology.

Functional and lifestyle medicine is clearly positioned to benefit from this intersection, but only if we can get our act together.

As James Maskell says,

---

## "It's about time we started acting like we're winning and not like we're losing"

---

I wrote this book to show you how to win at practicing functional medicine, so that you can create an extraordinary life for yourself and your patients.

## THE MOST IMPORTANT ADVICE I CAN OFFER

Before you embark on this journey or decide you're going to scale your practice, I want you to deeply reflect on what it is you truly want your practice to do for you, your family, and your community.

There is no sense in building a business that ruins your life and your relationships and robs you of your freedom.

I've missed many family events, milestone moments, and evening meals. There is no amount of money that can buy back any of those.

Remember:

---

*Making money should never cost you the things that money can't buy*

---

.As you start this journey, keep close to your heart and on your mind what is important to you.

When I lost everything, my car couldn't hug me and reassure me everything was going to be okay; it was my family that was there for me.

One of the reasons I'm writing this book is you can have more dinners with your family.

As Dave Gambrill says,

---

*"Build a business around your life, instead of a life around your business"*

---

## THE FIRST FIFTY

Functional medicine training is very important, but nothing trumps the compliance of your patients. The best clinical experience you will ever get will come from experience with *compliant* patients. Your clinical confidence hinges on the ability of your patients to comply with your recommendations.

---

*No matter how much training you have or how many degrees and certificates you have hanging on your wall, the patient will ultimately determine the outcome*

---

Screening your patients from the very beginning, ensuring that they are going to comply with your recommendations, and setting up realistic goals for them to accomplish will be critical to their outcomes.

By carefully evaluating the patients you are bringing into your office, you can ensure that the training you have gets implemented.

There is nothing more frustrating than patients who are not following your recommendations because they're not getting results, and they're giving your practice a bad name.

Your first 50 to 100 patients will set the tone in your practice, determine your clinical confidence, and affect your ability to advance and scale your business.

If your patients are noncompliant, you will begin to question your training, seek more conferences, and incorrectly blame yourself for the lack of outcomes.

The greatest tragedy in all this is that you blame yourself instead of addressing the real issue, noncompliant patients!

When you start your practice, you're much more likely to qualify patients based on finances, because you're likely challenged by finances early on. My best advice to you is to *only* work with your ideal clients, because your practice will grow exponentially instead of incrementally.

Working with your ideal clients means that you always get excellent outcomes, you feel more rewarded knowing patients are getting better under your care, your confidence increases, you deliver more value, and your charge a fair price. Sounds like a pretty sweet deal!

---

*Screen your patients to produce a better outcome instead of screening them to make a higher income.*

---

## I'm New. Should I Hire a Mentor?

Many practitioners fall into the trap of thinking that their success hinges on their clinical skill set. While your knowledge is valuable, it doesn't replace experience.

I refer to any training as *just in case* information. You take in tons of information in the event you might need it someday on the magical patient that read the book!

The best training for learning to implement this information is mentorship. The more certainty you have in your actions, the faster your practice will grow.

Think of it this way: You'd be much better off having someone sitting next to you when you learn how to drive a car or fly a plane versus someone teaching you about it in a book.

Clinical and practice mentorship provides you with a valuable sounding board so that you have even more certainty in growing your practice and more confidence in your clinical recommendations.

When you feel lost you slow down, you lose momentum and in many cases return to your comfort zone.

Imagine being able to get real-time feedback so that you can take the right steps from the very beginning. It's easier to move a wall on the blueprint rather than after the house is built.

As someone who made every mistake in the book, I can tell you that one of the biggest was not hiring a mentor sooner.

My mentors have been instrumental in my success, because they often see a potential in me that I did not know existed. My mentors have saved me millions of dollars and years of my life by steering me clear of danger.

I can only imagine how much bigger my business would have grown had I hired a mentor from the very beginning.

When hiring a mentor, be sure to work with someone who has all areas of their life dialed in, not just someone who knows how to achieve business success.

---

## If all you want to do is make money, all you will do is make money

---

Mentorship is the closest thing that I can of think of to a time machine. When you work with a mentor, you're leveraging all the time they've put into their craft as well as their relationships.

Mentorship can be one of the more important decisions you make to determine your personal and professional success.

There are several amazing functional medicine mentorships out there. I suggest that you call around and find one that suits your goals and core values.

Towards the end of this book, I've put together a self-assessment to help you decide if coaching and mentorship are right for you.

# PERSONAL GROWTH

# THE POWER OF LANGUAGE

A few years ago, I learned an important lesson from my mentor
Dr. Gilles Lamarche, who learned this lesson from Dr. Wayne Dyer.

The English language is one of the most confusing languages.
Semantically it's terrible, and I truly believe that this is done with the
intention to confuse the masses (but that's a different book).

As a father, I've had to become hyperaware of the English
language only to realize how confusing it is. Some words sound the
same but have entirely different meanings (buy, bye, by), while
some words actually imply the opposite of the speaker's intention
(incredible, unbelievable).

Moving forward, if you ever hear someone using the word
*incredible* to describe something, please correct them immediately
as their language is sabotaging their credibility at a subconscious
level. They have no idea that they are even doing it!

Other words to become hyperconscious of are *don't, can't, won't*.
The human brain cannot think in negatives. So, when you say, "I
don't want to fail in practice," you are vibrationally saying, "I want to
fail in practice." There is no such thing as a negative vibration.
Keep your language positive to create the circumstances of your
choosing.

I suggest that you give your staff and close friends permission to
correct you when you use the words listed above, it will be an
important lesson in your personal development. You will be
shocked at the number of times people use the wrong words in
dialogue.

This concept is known as semantic sabotage.

## THE IMPORTANCE OF OUR THOUGHTS

First, there was the word.

Language (verbal and body) is one of the most important aspects of human interaction. Words create vibration and vibration creates the organization of matter. Not all vibration can be heard, but that doesn't mean it does not exist.

Thoughts are high-level vibrations that we cannot hear. However, they are capable of organizing matter in the same accordance to their frequency. Therefore, our thoughts are critical, much more powerful than the words we use.

Be extremely mindful concerning what you think about with respect to every area of your life.

Your brain is like a wireless supercomputer that is conducting billions of processes and propagating complex messages into the world around you.

Think about all the times you thought of someone, and they called you or emailed you a few seconds later. There are no coincidences; there is only organization to matter.

How you organize your thoughts is how your life will organize in correspondence. Your thoughts are projected into the world to create your reality.

Just like a computer can erase and retype, you can do the same. If you find yourself thinking negatively, immediately change your thoughts to being positive. It's okay to make adjustments like this, just like it's okay to make changes on your computer screen.

Think of your thoughts like driving; pay close attention and make adjustments as required to navigate to where you want to go.

Just like driving, it's important to keep your focus on where you want to get to versus all the places you are not trying to get to.

Focus clearly on what you want and put your foot on the gas. Stay steadfast and consistent in your focus and watch amazing circumstances manifest from your thought vibrations.

When you learn to tap into this gift (available to all), amazing opportunities present themselves.

It's more important to know what you want before you know how you are going to get there.

Seemingly random circumstances can speed up any timeline you have in mind.

Trust this process, it has served me tremendously. In fact, this is one of the most important lessons I can possibly teach you.

## SCARCITY VS. ABUNDANCE

In my opinion, one of the biggest factors holding back the functional medicine movement is the mindset of practitioners. There is no shortage of patients that need your help or services. In fact, the people that need your expertise continue to grow in exponential numbers. The entire population is getting sicker due to a variety of factors.

People are not in pursuit of more medications or more surgeries. They are in search of root cause resolution and to deeply connect with someone with regard to their health.

Every time someone leaves the doctor's office or hospital, they probably wish they were in your office. Except we have one major issue, they don't even know you exist!

The mindset that we approach the problem with will determine the heights of our impact and success. There are two mindsets that we must become aware of so that we can consciously control our behaviors and thoughts to correspond with the outcomes we are trying to create. These two mindsets are the scarcity mindset and the abundance mindset.

Before you continue reading, it's important to pause and reflect on your mindset. Many times, this mindset comes from deep subconscious programming from well-intentioned parents and teachers. If your parents had a scarcity mindset, it *will* show up later in your life to create a worldview filled with limiting beliefs and corresponding behaviors, which will lead to corresponding outcomes.

This information comes from a talk by Dan Sullivan at Genius Network in front of the most successful business owners and innovators in the world, so pay close attention.

## The scarcity mindset

There are three characteristics of the scarcity mindset that you must become aware of and address:

1. **Zero-sum game** – This leads to the ideation that if I have something, it's because I took it from someone else. Kind of like a poker game, except in reality there is an infinite reservoir of chips.

2. **Resources are being depleted** – while this is the theme of most new reports and articles these days, there is a key distinction that we must make. There is only one real resource and that this human ingenuity. It's human ingenuity that turns oil into empires, that turns mountains into mines, that turns trees into paper. Human ingenuity scales with the population and enables humans to create new resources through their amazing brain power!

3. **The world is unfair** – a person who buys into this worldview will live in a constant state of resentment, because they think that their world is conspiring against them. They are often envious of others; and everywhere they look, they see a problem.

It's hard to imagine the catastrophic results that this worldview can create, so let's focus on the way you should channel your energy.

## The abundance mindset

The abundance mindset turns your brain into a powerful tool to create whatever reality you desire. Sounds like a big promise, but you're going to have to trust me and thousands of successful entrepreneurs that think this way.

There are three characteristics of the abundance mindset that you must become aware of:

1. **Exponentials** – people with an abundance mindset think in exponentials instead of increments. An example would be the difference between a practice trying to grow their audience by 10 percent vs. 10 times. A good case study would be when a practitioner does a live presentation vs. one that records the presentation and streams it to thousands of people all over the world. A person of abundance realizes that there are a thousand times more people who are not in the room that need their help.

2. **Resourcefulness** – A person with an abundant mindset is resourceful and knows where you find answers and when to ask other for help. This line of thinking results in a problem-solving mindset vs. a problem-identifying mindset.

3. **Gratitude** – There are two types of gratitude, reactive and proactive. When we *appreciate* something or someone, their value *appreciates*. It is impossible to experience abundance if you do not have gratitude. If you ever encounter a situation where you are mad at someone or a situation, simply think of the reasons you are grateful for it and figure out how to tap into your resources (ideas, money, relationships, creativity).

This should be a good starting point for you to carefully evaluate your worldview. If necessary, I suggest that you seek the required help to overcome a scarcity mindset. This mindset will spill into every area of your life, such as relationships, investments, businesses, and all other circumstances.

## THE MOST ESSENTIAL SKILL TO DEVELOP

The ability to speak publicly is the most effective skill I have ever developed. The ability to speak in front of a crowd and get them to make a decision is an invaluable tool, especially as a functional medicine practitioner.

My public speaking ability has been developed and honed over the course of many years, delivering hundreds of workshops in my community and on professional stages.

The best way to get better at public speaking is to do more talks. The more talks you do, the better you will get. You will get better every single time you speak in front of a crowd.

Public speaking is one of the top fears people have. And if the idea of public speaking is making you nervous right now, I have only proved my point.

Communication is one of the most important skills that you have, and the ability to effectively communicate your message to your patients or your prospects is going to be critical in determining your success as a practitioner and the success of your practice.

Becoming a better speaker has enabled me to serve a thousand times more than I could have ever imagined. It's taken me to some of the most amazing places on the planet and has enabled me to connect with some the most influential leaders from several industries.

# HERO'S JOURNEY

First and foremost, I strongly suggest you carefully plot out your own hero's journey so you can connect much more effectively with your audience.

Stories are what connect people, not facts. Facts are great for shock value, but not great for connection. If you want to connect with your audience, be vulnerable. Share your story. Share your struggle.

If you're a functional medicine practitioner, chances are this is a second career for you. You probably had your life transformed through the journey you were on, and functional medicine helped you in some way.

Be vulnerable with how you got where you are right now, and this will make you much more credible. Patients will realize you can be empathetic to their concerns and that you understand what it's like to be on the other side of the desk.

Make this part of every single talk you do. It never gets old, and most people will be hearing it for the first time. This is where you build the majority of your connection.

Some practitioners have mistakenly shied away from their hero's journey, missing an opportunity to deeply connect with their audience and share their story.

For more resources on creating your hero's journey go to www.perfectpracticebook.com

## WHO IS YOUR UNFAIR ADVANTAGE?

Every practitioner or entrepreneur needs an *unfair advantage*. You need someone in your life who is going to support you and help you make the best decisions possible for you, for your business, and for the people you serve in your practice and your community.

My unfair advantage is my wife. My wife has been with me through thick and thin. She has supported me in every decision I have made. She has been there for me when I needed her the most and provided a solid sounding board for me to bounce ideas off of.

**Who is your unfair advantage?**

It might be a colleague, it might be a mentor, it might be your spouse, it might be a relative, or it might be your son or daughter.

This person should be someone who is close to you, someone who is invested in your best life, and someone who can be brutally honest with you and tell you when you need to straighten up your act.

Your unfair advantage is the person in your life that will transform the course of your life and determine the heights of success that you will reach.

## WORK–LIFE INTEGRATION

As an entrepreneur, it's tough to achieve "work–life balance," especially if you're doing your life's work.

I have personally found over the years that it is much easier to have work–life integration.

For those of you that follow me online, you must wonder how I (and others) create so much content and seem to do so many other cool things.

Well, here's the secret. I have a great team, *and* I work a few minutes of every hour instead of working several hours in continuum and then shutting everything down.

You see, I truly love helping thousands of people when I create new content. Who doesn't? What I also love is being with my family. Again, who doesn't?

By having an integrative strategy, I get the best of both worlds. I can check email a few times a day, post periodically as an idea comes to me, and still be hanging out with my friends and family. It's the best of both worlds. Work doesn't pile up, people appreciate the responsiveness, and I feel in full control of my life.

If you don't like a cluttered inbox, piles of to-dos, patients (and opportunities) waiting to hear from you, I suggest that you consider an integration strategy.

It does take self-control to stay on top of things without getting sucked into your computer or phone, but the payoff is worth the effort.

## Honoring My Mentors and Influencers

Over the years, I have had the pleasure of personally working with some very influential people. Influential doesn't mean that the person is famous; it simply means that they have had a profound impact on my life. I want to take a moment to honor some of my mentors for their dedication to their craft and their willingness to take me under their wings.

In no particular order, I would like to thank:

> - Dr. Ron Grisanti
> - Dr. Peter Osborne
> - Dr. Fuad Amer
> - Dr. Shawn Williams
> - Dr. Matthew Loop
> - Dr. Dan Kalish
> - Dr. Gilles Lamarche
> - Dr. James Chestnut
> - Dr. Ritesh Patel
> - Dr. Jared Seigler
> - Dr. Ricky Brar
> - Manu Singh
> - Tibi Murariu
> - Peter Jenkins
> - Fabio Soares
> - Cyd Alper-Sedgwick
> - James Maskell
> - Gabe Hoffman
> - Uli Iserloh
> - Charles Poliquin
> - Jordan Bokser
> - Mike Mutzel
> - Alex Charfen
> - Joe Polish
> - Rick Jones

## BOOKS TO READ

Over the past 6 years, I've read over 200 books and counting. The secret to my high consumption is an app called Audible. Audible is available on your smartphone and enables you to listen to virtually any book on your phone.

I listened to my first audiobook during a drive from Toronto to Cincinnati, *Crush It!*, by Gary Vaynerchuk. The book was suggested to me by my friend Manu Singh, so I bought it. The length of the book was the length of the drive, so it worked out perfectly.

Less than a week later, I started my first blog! That book started my online career, because it inspired me to leverage technology and reach the masses.

My blog was really simple; it answered a question I got after every nutrition consult, "What do you eat?"

I started to share recipes of the meals that my wife would prepare for our family. It was a simple concept that just really seemed to take off with my Facebook friends, because it added tremendous value to their lives.

Think about that. A book changed my life and my practice and has inspired me to write this book for you. Books can be very subjective, and the list keeps changing for me, so I thought I would share some important books to start with on the following page.

When you go to www.perfectpracticebook.com, I share a special link where you can get two free books on Audible to get started.

## My suggested listening list

1. *The Bhagavad Gita: A Guide for Westerners* – Jack Hawley
2. *The Go-Giver* – David Mann
3. *The Art of Exceptional Living* – Jim Rohn
4. *Warrior of Light* – Paulo Coelho
5. *The Biology of Belief* – Dr. Bruce Lipton
6. *Crush it!* – Gary Vaynerchuk
7. *The Four Agreements* – Don Miguel Ruiz
8. *How Successful People Think* – John Maxwell
9. *Steve Jobs* – Walter Isaacson
10. *Change Your Thoughts, Change Your Life* – Dr. Wayne Dyer
11. *Making Money Is Killing Your Business* – Chuck Blakeman
12. *Insanely Simple* – Ken Segall
13. *Men Are from Mars, Women Are from Venus* – Dr. John Gray
14. *Start with Why* – Simon Sinek
15. *The E-Myth* – Michael Gerber
16. *Zero to One* – Peter Thiel
17. *Secrets of The Close* – Zig Ziglar
18. *Leap First* – Seth Godin
19. *Autobiography of A Yogi* – Paramahansa Yogananda
20. *Do the Work* – Steven Pressfield

## Books to purchase:

1. *Expert Secrets* – Russel Brunson
2. *Think and Grow Rich* – Napoleon Hill
3. *How Social Media Made Me Rich and How It Can Do the Same For You* – Matthew Loop
4. *Positive Personality Profiles* – Robert Rohm

Please visit www.perfectpracticebook.com to get the most up-to-date list

# PRACTICE PRINCIPLES

## THE BEST WAY TO SET UP YOUR PRACTICE

In functional medicine, there is very little capital cost involved. Most of the costs involved in functional medicine are devoted to training and skill development.

One of the key advantages that we have as entrepreneurs in this new space is we do not require a lot of equipment to run our practices. In fact, all you need is an office for consultations.

If you are doing telemedicine, all you need is a computer and a video camera to consult with your patient. It's never been a better time to be alive!

The overhead for functional medicine is unusually low for a healthcare practice. This is our unfair advantage. We not only provide a higher level of service and make our patients' dollars go much further, we carve out more profit, especially starting out in business.

Many businesses take many years to recover their initial investment. Your practice can be profitable within the first month using the method I am going to discuss.

My suggestion is to locate a smart office near your home and start inquiring about leasing opportunities. This has been the secret sauce to our immediate success and liquidity as a business.

I've grown two successful practices out of smart office settings and have been profitable from the first month.

## SMART OFFICES

When I started looking for office space to open my functional medicine practice, I thought I would have to go the traditional route of leasing space, building it out, and signing a five- to ten-year contract.

I would then have to furnish the place, buying furniture and the necessary equipment. I would also have to set up the phone lines and the Internet, choose the finishing and the carpeting, pay an electrical bill, and pay an Internet bill every month.

The costs pile up very, very quickly.

During my initial search, I encountered an office setup called Regus. The Regus saleslady asked me to connect with a furniture saleslady to choose the furniture for my office.

It turned out the furniture saleslady was a good friend of mine. Based on my needs, she suggested that I look at a "smart office" location instead.

This is a smart office setup where everything is included in one payment. It includes your own private office, secretaries to answer your phones for you and greet your prospective patients or clients, your furniture, your Internet, and your phone line.

Everything is rolled into one payment.

When I opened my practice, I was only paying a thousand dollars a month to have an office fully staffed, fully furnished, and fully taken care of.

Because I was mainly providing a consulting service, I did not need anything more than that. This setup forced me to develop and implement technology that would educate my patients and inform them about what I do, without having to have the front desk answer my phone.

It forced me to create online scheduling for my practice, so I didn't have to rely on somebody else answering my patients' questions and scheduling for me.

Certainly, they could have done it, but I decided that I wanted to leverage technology as best I could, since patients are usually searching online for answers when the office is not open anyway.

The smart office eliminated the headache of having to hire a person to manage the front desk, worry about whether they're going to show up or not, and worry about whether the phone was going to be answered or not.

It also provided a space to practice where all the maintenance and cleaning was taken care of. I could just show up, and everything was done for me.

It also provided me with additional space to host conferences. We had a teaching kitchen within the space to host our patients for cooking and food preparation workshops. It was the perfect setup.

It was amazing I found a space like this to help me get my practice off the ground and become immediately profitable. This eliminated much of the stress that most practitioners have when starting a business, and there was almost no risk. If I wanted to shut my office down, I just had to give a 60-day notice.

Smart offices are also known as co-working spaces, so be sure to search a variety of terms to find one close to you.

Most towns will have similar options or shared-space locations. If you live in a big enough town, these should be popping up everywhere. You might be sharing your common space with other professionals such as attorneys or lawyers.

# Enhancing Your Client Experience

One of the ways we help enhance our client experience is by recording how-to videos. In these videos, we explain lab testing instructions that walk the patient through the exact steps.

Chances are if you do that in the office, by the time the patient gets home they are probably not going to remember most of what you told them.

If you can share a video that goes through every detail that they need to know and post it to a page with the rest of your videos on how to do lab testing, you will significantly minimize the number of questions that people have.

To provide the best experience for your clients, I also encourage periodic check-ins. These check-ins can be done manually, or can be done automatically if you have an autoresponder.

I use specific extensions like Boomerang for Chrome, which allows me to send an email out at a prespecified time. This means I can send an email out two weeks from today to my patient.

This ensures the follow-up will be sent, it keeps the dialog and engagement going, and the patient feels supported at the same time.

When patients join our practice, we provide them with as much information as they need to take the next steps. Try not to overload them with everything that they need to know in one visit. Remember you have several months to work with them and get them feeling well.

The last thing that you want is for them to feel overwhelmed. You want them to walk away with one to three things that they need to do before their next appointment, and you need to hold them accountable to those things.

If you overwhelm people, they will not have a good experience. They will have more questions than you can handle, which will come in constantly and bog down your system.

When patients become overwhelmed, they often don't do anything. Keep the momentum going with simple action steps and supporting videos or literature for them.

# WHAT ARE THE ADVANTAGES OF CASE FEES?

There is an ongoing debate about whether practitioners should charge a case fee for their services or if they should charge a pay-as-you-go model.

Over the years, I have found that charging patients a case fee works better for both parties. Not only does the practitioner have better cash flow, but the patient gets a more comprehensive and complete service.

Patients who pay in advance are much more committed to the process. Patients who are committed drastically lower your mental and financial overhead.

It is important that the individual follow through with your recommendations if you are going to be putting in significant effort to crack a person's case open, determine their underlying mechanisms, and create a plan to get them well again.

If your staff is constantly having to follow up with patients to get them to come in or chase people down to render services, this creates a lot of frustration for both you and your team.

More importantly, patients do not get the results they were hoping for and that you know you could deliver. By lowering this overhead significantly, it enables you and your team to focus on what really matters: patients wanting to get better, patients wanting to transform their lives, and patients who are committed to their best life.

By charging a case fee, you are also enabling yourself to recover the costs that go into prepping a case, interpreting lab results, and completing all the paperwork that goes on behind the scenes.

Charging a case fee also helps you recover the cost of acquisition. In many instances, if you are practicing on a pay-as-you-go model, it might take several visits until you recover the costs of acquiring the patient. Not a good situation!

This means that if a patient only comes in a couple of times, you have actually lost money working with them. Yes, we are in the business of helping people, but we are also in the business of staying in business.

It is important you have a strategy that allows you to engage with people who are committed to your process, who are going to follow through with your process, who are going to get results through the process, and patients who refer others just like them.

By having a case fee, you are able to deliver a tremendous amount of value and additional services since your overhead drops dramatically, and your cash flow improves significantly.

Check out what's included in our Living Proof Essentials Program if you're looking for inspiration. www.lpiessentials.com

# WORLD-CLASS EXPERIENCES

Charging a case fee also allows you to add additional services and enables you to provide a world-class experience for your clients. Patients have been to plenty of practitioners, and they have had plenty of empty promises.

Not only are they looking for results, but your clients are also looking for a world-class experience coupled with those results. From what I have seen in my practice, patients who get a world-class experience generally tend to get better results.

If someone does not get a world-class experience, you can put your best effort into their case, but their results will often be as lackluster as their experience.

Additional services that we can offer our clients are email access, video lab interpretations, group classes, exclusive webinars, exclusive offers, and many other bonuses.

We offer these as part of our entire program, rather than having patients pay for every single service they receive. By grouping or bundling services and having your clients pay in advance, it significantly lowers your financial and mental overhead. This frees up your staff to do what is really important, which is deliver world-class service to the clients that are committed to your care.

It enables you to get amazing results with patients because you are able to see them through their course of care with the right number of visits and the right number of touchpoints. You are able to go above and beyond the traditional pay-as-you-go model.

When discussing why you charge a case fee to your patients, simply point out the benefits to the patient and the practice.

Let them know that your staff can focus on client care instead of chasing them down for follow-up appointments.

Let them know that you and your practitioners don't get bogged down by patients that are not fully committed to the care it's going to take to get them well.

It takes a seriously committed patient to get well, and you're going to have to be able to do the job that's required to make it happen. In the end, it will be your reputation on the line, so at least be certain you can do your job.

## Automation vs. Personalization

It's attractive to think that we can have a computer do a bunch of mundane tasks for us such as sending emails, automated education, and flowing patients through a funnel, but remember that people are looking for a personal touch.

Your practice must focus on mastering automation but also mastering the personalization of the patient experience. Patients will refer based on their experience before they refer based on results. In fact, it's not unusual for patients to refer others solely based on their experience.

I would strongly argue that the user experience influences patient outcomes more than anything else. Trust me, coffee tastes different when it is served with a smile versus an attitude.

Remember you have full control over the user experience but almost no control over the ultimate outcome (which your patient creates for themselves), so it's important that the user experience gets special attention.

There are several ways that you can significantly improve the impression you make and experience you create for your client.

Over the years, we've tried several different ideas. Here are the ones that we use today:

1. Welcome package mailed with branded intention jar, mug, and thank you card
2. Gratitude Journal at second appointment
3. Signed birthday cards
4. Referral thank you cards
5. Weekly Q&A in Facebook group
6. Welcome call and check-ins
7. Live patient education events and workshops
8. Patient appreciation events
9. Bringing in guest speakers
10. Surveying our patients to improve our process

As simple as many of these ideas sound, it's rare that any practice is doing even a few of these. Starting out it might seem like a lot of work, but so is constantly trying to get new patients because you're not getting enough referrals.

When you create a unique experience for your patients, you elevate yourself from being a price-based commodity to being the go-to choice for your community.

*It's easier to get 50 people to refer one person a month than it is to get one person to bring in 50 new patients a month.*

*Create an extraordinary experience for your patients, and they will reward you with endless referrals and rapid scale.*

## THE BEST WAY TO BUILD YOUR TEAM

Your staff is one of the most important determinants of your practice's success, and it is important the people you hire are fully aligned with the mission statement of your practice.

Anyone in your office has the capability to make or break your practice. It is critical to hire people who share your core values from a service standpoint, but also from a financial mindset standpoint.

---

*Your team must understand the value that you deliver into your community and understand the costs associated with running a business.*

---

As you know, there is more to it than meets the eye.

One of the most effective things that we have done when hiring is to only hire patients whose lives have been transformed through our program. This has proven to be instrumental in their success on the team. Your entire team has to fully embrace your vision and mission. If they don't it will hold the whole practice back.

Someone who has invested in your program will have a much easier time supporting others in their decision.

Someone who has not transformed through the process cannot genuinely and passionately encourage others. It's easy for you to "sell" functional medicine when it changed your life!

If you have a passionate group of people that complement each other, share core values, and have had a transformative experience with your business, you can only begin to imagine the possibilities.

Much of the emotional stress in running a business comes from staff. Thankfully, I've been blessed with an amazing team of passionate and talented people.

If you're planning to build a team around you, I suggest getting to know yourself first. Having an honest self-assessment of your personality and communication style; you can build a team that complements your strengths and vulnerabilities.

I strongly suggest three self-assessment tools to get started:

1. DISC communication style
2. Kolbe – A
3. 5 Love Languages

You can learn more about these tools, test yourself and your team at www.perfectpracticebook.com

When starting out, the first person you hire will be critical to your success. Therefore, hiring the right person, someone who is fully aligned with your vision and core values, is very important. I cannot stress this enough.

In my case, my wife was my first (paid and unpaid) employee. She is my perfect complement; her support is what makes all of this possible.

It turns out our personality testing even proves we are a great complement to each other!

I would suggest that you immediately take the testing above to get a better sense of yourself and for identifying your perfect first team member to grow your practice with.

As my team has grown, we have created a chart for easy access to our team's personality, communication, and action styles. At a quick glance, I know exactly who is best suited for each role, project, or task.

Each team member is placed in a role and assigned tasks that suit their strengths. This process might seem tedious at first, but it only takes a few minutes to collect information that is transformative to both the team member and your practice.

# You Are Only as Good as Your Team

Your team is absolutely critical, because they are going to deliver the care your company is providing.

Because your company is also going to be community facing, it is important these individuals have a positive relationship and impression within the community.

You want to be sure that you are checking out the social media pages of these individuals to make sure that they represent your brand properly.

The team that you hire, when done correctly, will help your practice flourish. Always keep in mind that people will come and go. People will move on, and it is your duty to keep your team and mission in full alignment.

*A great litmus test will be if you are getting emails at least once a month from people asking if they can work for you. This tells you that the energy your team exudes makes your office a desirable place to do meaningful work*

Many people will tell you to hire slow and fire fast, and this can be good advice. My experience has been "listen to your gut." Your gut will always steer you right.

If you are looking to hire someone for a specific role or a specific task that is critical and vital to your business, the best job interview is not talking to that person. The best job interview is giving them a task, having them complete that task, and then observing the quality of the work that that person provides.

If you need someone to play a technical role, but they have no technical background or they are not willing to figure it out themselves in a YouTube era, chances are that person is not going to be very resourceful.

You always want to hire people that take work off your plate, not add more to it.

---

*Only hire a person who has been transformed by your services, works towards the same vision, has an abundance mindset, complements your skills, and is resourceful.*

---

Sound impossible?

Just remember you will always attract who you are.

# FOREVER GRATITUDE JOURNALS

Gratitude is an essential part of healing. It is so important we set an example of our gratitude for our patients and for those who do business with us.

One of the ways we do this is by offering every single one of our patients a gratitude journal. We specifically use the Five-Minute Journal.

One of the key features of our gratitude journals is they never run out; we provide an infinite gratitude journal to our clients. This means that when they bring their journal back to us, filled out, we will supply them with a brand new one for them to keep (and they get to keep their original one too).

If you have someone filling out a gratitude journal every morning and every evening, guess who they are thinking of every time they open up that book? They are thinking of you, and they are probably thinking of how amazing you have helped them feel.

They are probably thinking of people you could help on their journey as well. A gratitude journal is a great way to stay in contact with your best patients and allow them to experience the benefits of gratitude, but also the benefits of your ongoing relationship with them.

## ADDITIONAL TOUCH POINTS

Another way to stay in contact with your patients and support them on their journey is to share automated educational emails that are sent out to them once a week. You can time these automations and the content to correspond to where they would be on their journey.

This content can be videos you share, new recipes, clever ideas, or Ted Talks you think the patient should watch at this juncture in their journey. There could be a variety of things to help people along the way.

We share a book of the week with our patients. Our office reads one book every week, and this allows us to have great conversation and grow professionally and personally. Sharing the books you are reading might inspire your prospective patients and your current patients to read the same books and align with your growth and philosophy.

One of the highest touch points we provide, aside from our appointments, is live group presentations. We deliver in-person workshops. We also share them live on Facebook, where people can connect with like-minded people and discuss various topics.

These topics might include stress management, exercise, meditation, yoga, essential oils, group cooking classes, and a variety of other topics.

We survey our patients periodically to find out what they are most interested in. Group workshops can be an excellent platform for patients to bring their friends and family members who they might consider to be a good fit for the practice.

As a private practice, your goal is to provide exceptional service and care. Unfortunately, in the healthcare industry, good service is a rare offering.

You can easily set yourself apart by helping your patients feel supported, by helping them feel nurtured, by answering their questions before they even come up, and by answering questions live for them. This way they can feel engaged and connected to you, while you are leveraging and making the best use of your time, energy, and effort.

# MARKETING AND MESSAGING

# FUNDAMENTALS OF MARKETING YOUR PRACTICE

Your content should have three critical pillars. Everything that leaves your office should have these three pillars in place. These pillars are connection, action, and a measurable result.

## Pillar 1: Connection

When you connect with your audience, you understand their needs. You are able to put yourself in their shoes so you can better understand the questions they might have, the concerns they might have, and the problems they are encountering.

It is important that you develop an instantaneous connection with people, so they become more engaged in your content.

## Pillar 2: Action

It is important that you provide your audience with some sort of action step so they can feel an instantaneous benefit from the connection they have made with you.

You might have them opt in for a free one-week shopping list and accompanying meal plan. You can then capture their email address and put them into your customer relationship management platform to further nurture and escalate them through your onboarding funnels.

Make sure you give them content that allows them to take instant action, not something that bogs them down.

If you give them something impossible to do, guess what? They are not going to do it, and they are going to assume that being a patient in your office is extremely difficult and challenging.

They may never engage with you ever again. Make sure you meet people where they are on the journey.

**Pillar 3: Result**

You should be able to quantify in some way the outcomes of your marketing efforts. Facebook and Google provide us with amazing analytical tools to be able to understand the return on our investment.

Sometimes it can be very challenging to know exactly where people are coming from. They may have been following you through several sites and found you on several platforms. But maybe that last Facebook video that you did encouraged them to take action, or maybe it was a podcast that they just heard you on.

Some things are easier to track than others, but you can be quite certain that it's going to take multiple touch points before somebody becomes a patient at your office.

In fact, the more touch points they have, the better qualified they are, since they are more familiar with your message.

# A SEVEN-STEP MARKETING STRATEGY

Does your practice have a marketing strategy or is everything randomly strung together in the hopes that something sticks?

The following information comes from my mentor Pam Hendrickson, who worked alongside Tony Robbins for over 20 years.

## Step 1: Content mission

Your content mission statement affects everything you do. For example, our content mission statement is,

---

*to help transform functional medicine practices, help healers create and deliver world-class healthcare services that generate a meaningful profit, and help transform people's lives*

---

Everything we send out to people is going to keep our content mission statement in mind.

Here are some questions to ask:

> ➤ Does this content provide value for the defined avatar?
> ➤ Does it deliver the promise we are offering?
> ➤ Does it provide something meaningful as a result?

## Step 2: Break it down

The second step is to break your marketing down into three to five smaller goals.

Here are some examples:

> ➤ What are your goals with respect to your marketing?

- ➢ Are you looking for increased engagement on Facebook and YouTube or other social media platforms?
- ➢ Are you trying to grow your list by a certain percentage every month, quarter, or year?
- ➢ Are you creating compelling and consistent experiences for your online brand?
- ➢ Are you looking to establish yourself as an expert or a speaker and get hired for a certain number of engagements every year?

Have some sort of big picture metric of your marketing strategy.

## Step 3: Identify your target audience

The third step is to identify your target audience, by not only their demographics but also their psychographics.

Psychographics provide a deep, emotional alignment with the patient. The more specific you can get with the patient, the better your marketing efforts will respond.

## Step 4: Your core message

The fourth step is to identify your core message. Do you have a certain way that you want your audience to feel? Be sure to share your core message with all of your branding and marketing.

Your core message may include:

- ➢ compassion
- ➢ empathy
- ➢ a continuous sense of growth
- ➢ improvement
- ➢ learning
- ➢ partnership
- ➢ accountability

Make sure that if these are your core values, they come through in everything that you do.

66

# Step 5: Where will you reach people?

There are two components Pam discusses: the bricks in your business and the feathers in your business.

Your bricks are your meatier content that will be the more meaningful and deeper engagements with your audience. These are going to include things like Facebook LIVE videos, emails, or even an app you might have. They might also include webinars or blog posts that your audience engages in.

Your feathers are your social media content. These might be articles, ideas, short videos, or content that you share online. These are not the foundation of your content, but they are nice additions.

Make sure you have a balance between bricks and feathers in your business.

## Step 6: Measure

You want to have some way to measure the consumption of the content to be sure it's moving the needle in the right direction. You can measure how many people are sharing the content, how many leads are signing up for your autoresponders or your landing pages, and what the conversion rate is.

Conversions into your programs, or sales of your programs, would also be important to measure.

## Step 7: Create a content calendar

You'll want to plan your events every quarter if possible. Be open to changing the topic of the event, if need be. You can decide as the month gets closer and closer.

You might change direction, but have something in your calendar so you're booking the rest of your events, your life, and your travel around those hard dates in your calendar.

It is important for you to have a quarterly vision of what is going on in your business if you are playing the long game.

You do not want to be living workshop to workshop in your practice!

My suggestion to you is to sit down with your team and review your current marketing strategy to be sure it fulfills the criteria outlined above.

Once you have the right framework and intention set up, your marketing efforts will become a lot easier to implement, measure, and benefit from.

Remember it's going to take several touch points for someone to become a patient, so keep your marketing efforts consistent, be sure to play the long game, and remember,

---

## *Consistency carves canyons*

---

## COMMON MARKETING MISTAKES

I get it. You're not a marketer. But that doesn't mean you should be a bad marketer, either.

There are two mistakes people make when marketing. The first mistake is they never ask for a sale. They never ask their prospects to take any action, and by doing this, you are essentially training your followers to not buy anything!

This can potentially be a huge problem. You are training your audience to think you are constantly going to give them information without asking for anything in return.

The second mistake people make is the exact opposite. They ask too much, they ask too early, or they ask the wrong questions at the wrong time.

It is important that you find this sacred balance with your audience and your avatar. Segment your list based on the level of engagement and where these people are on their journey towards health.

You would never ask someone to marry you the first time you meet them. In fact, there are probably lots of people out there that you would not want to do business with.

The idea is to get people on base and engaged with your content. Make compelling offers periodically to properly condition your audience that not everything is FREE!

## THE AVATAR PARADOX

"What is an avatar?" you ask.

An avatar is your ideal client. When you think of your ideal client, think of every dimension of this individual.

Think of their health challenges, their personal challenges, and their emotional challenges. Think of what kind of car they drive, what neighborhood they live in, what type of work they do, what type of relationships they have, what level of education they have, what level of income they have, the proximity to your clinic, the knowledge level of this individual in the topic of specialty that you're in, the people that they might follow on social media, the podcasts that they might listen to, the type of clothing and brands they might use, etc.

You want to get as detailed and granular about your avatar as possible. Your avatar is the backbone of your business. One thing that many practitioners forget is that it is not only important for you to identify your avatar and attract your perfect client into your office, but it is important for you to realize that the client who is looking for a practitioner also has an avatar in mind. The patient's avatar of their ideal practitioner has to resemble who you are as well.

This is known as the avatar paradox.

---

Are you the avatar that your avatar is looking for?

---

# DO I NEED A NICHE?

One of the challenges functional medicine practitioners face is that they are equipped with the tools to help virtually any chronic condition.

Not a bad problem to have except when it comes to your marketing. You'll have a hard time marketing a workshop or webinar to anyone and everyone.

Before you pigeonhole yourself into a niche, I think it's important to know your audience. The best type of condition to work with is the very condition that you overcame using functional and lifestyle medicine.

If you overcame thyroid disease, digestive issues, or joint pain for example, who better to help others with the same issue.

It will be so much easier for you to relate and connect with your prospective patients, and you will build a deeper relationship with them. Many people visit a specialist that has never experienced the very conditions they specialize in. Their experience is not first hand. Nothing matches first-hand experience.

Your marketing becomes a cinch when you can say, "let me show you the exact principles I used to overcome XYZ condition."

There is a downside to working with people who already have a diagnosis: They have likely been struggling for many years with their issues before finding you.

In order for someone to find your niche practice, they have to know what their problem is. It's a catch-22.

As a word of caution, don't work with a particular audience just because other practitioners have busy practices with that niche.

If you study anyone who is at the top of their game, their practice niche is related to their personal story. Working with others who have faced similar challenges as you also helps boost your confidence, because you can both relate better with each other.

I've worked with thyroid patients, patients with digestive issues, autoimmunity, etc.; but to be honest, my greatest fulfillment comes from working with practitioners trying to build their practices. This is an area that I have spent an extraordinary amount of time and money on figuring out.

## YOUR SIGNATURE SERIES

Your signature series is a suite of digital products that represent your brand offering. These products are designed to work together in an escalating fashion to serve every member of society that needs to be able to tap into your core message.

By offering escalating products and services you can help people at various levels of their journey and income level. Let's face it. We'll never be able to help everyone, but that's no reason to create an inferior product.

Think of Apple in this case. All their products share the same core value and integrate very nicely together, thus enhancing the user experience and maintaining brand loyalty and appeal across many populations.

The first in this series of products should be your signature talk. You signature talk can be delivered live, as a podcast, or as a webinar. This talk should include an introduction to your core values and mission. It should compel listeners to take action.

My signature talk is, The Doctor of the Future (Is the Patient). My core message of patient-empowered root cause medicine shines through and drives people to my signature opt-in.

My signature opt-in further demonstrates my core values by showing people how to take better care of themselves. The program is completely free (but transformative). Check it out here: www.30in30.org.

Once people have gone through that program, you may invite them to a live workshop or webinar that goes a little bit deeper or offers them the opportunity to join your signature online course.

This remains hands-off for you but might include a group call periodically. An eight-week course can be priced at about $249–$499.

You can check out my signature online course, The Doctor of the Future, here: http://bit.ly/lpidotf.

Next is your signature program. This is your highest level of engagement and reserved for your most qualified clients. These are clients that you are going to spend time with over the next few months.

To learn more about our signature program, called The Essentials, go here: www.lpiessentials.com.

Through your signature series of digital and personal services, you can serve any audience (with any budget) and help move their health in the right direction.

# ANALOGIES TO EXPLAIN FUNCTIONAL MEDICINE

Analogies are an easy way for us to communicate complex relationships. By using concepts that are already accepted, applying an analogy to connect the two typically results in some significant paradigm shifts.

I'm sharing some simple analogies that you can start with to help communicate functional medicine to your patients, family, or colleagues.

## 1. The Car, the Driver, and the Environment

If you put rocket fuel in your car, does that make you a better driver?

If you put the most expensive fuel in your car, does that make you a better driver?

Focusing on becoming a better driver shifts the responsibility onto the patient.

If you saw a car in an accident, you would rarely ever blame the car itself; you would blame the weather or the driver.

Very rarely is your body the issue.

More often it is how you are taking care of your body.

How you are driving the car, whether the road conditions are bad, and whether the fuel is bad will all compromise your outcomes.

## 2. The Wilting Plant – Nature Is Not Negotiable

A plant has a requirement for how much sunlight and water it needs, and you cannot negotiate with the plant for what it needs to thrive.

You cannot compensate by giving the plant more water instead of more sunshine. The patient is the plant. If a patient's health is wilting, we must address the things they need to be healthy.

There are fundamental things you need to be healthy, and you cannot compromise on those. Giving a plant enough water but ignoring how much sunlight and soil it needs will never get the plant healthy.

### 3. The Gun

Our genetics load the gun, our thoughts aim the gun, and our environment pulls the trigger. We are all born in the image of perfection. The set of genetic cards you have was set up to thrive in optimal conditions.

People feel better on vacation, but being on vacation does not change your genetics. It changes your thoughts, focus, and environment.

### 4. Putting the Fire Out

Inflammation is a constant process that takes away from repair and healing. If one corner of your house is on fire, you're not going to be painting and decorating the other parts of the house.

You have to put the fire out and repair the damage from the fire first. You have to address the inflammation and repair the damage that has been done, and then you can look at building the body up and really healing.

### 5. Buckets Filling Up in the Yard

Imagine you have twenty buckets of all different sizes in your yard. These buckets represent the different systems in your body: thyroid, liver, GI, brain, skin, etc.

Now imagine, it begins to rain, and this rain represents stress and toxins. The buckets are all filling up with water at different rates. It's the same amount of rain that is falling across the yard, but the smaller buckets are going to fill up faster than the larger buckets.

The systems represented by the smaller buckets are more sensitive to environmental disruptions. The first bucket to fill up is usually the one that gets all the attention, but this ignores the fact that the other buckets are also filling up.

You have to address the cause of the buckets filling up; you have to address the fact that it is raining if you expect to get long-term outcomes.

## A Functional Medicine Consumer Guide

One of my mentors, Joe Polish, taught me about a very clever positioning tool that can transform your business's credibility by leaps and bounds.

A consumer guide is an excellent resource to help prospective patients realize the value of what you deliver.

I've written a guide called "A Consumer Guide to Choosing a Functional Medicine Practice." This 16-page guide is an outstanding resource for patients to receive either digitally or as a booklet.

The guide covers the hidden traps that patients should be conscious of when choosing a provider. It helps them become better detectives when researching your competitor. By knowing what questions to ask, the patient has a better consumer experience and is less likely to get taken advantage of.

Remember, we still care about people (even if they don't use our services). I hear way too often from patients, "I wish I met you five years ago before I blew my life savings." When a consumer has an experience like this, they become much more skeptical of the whole profession. The last thing this movement needs is patients who question everything but are asking all the wrong questions.

By using the guide, you leverage your role on the patient's journey and essentially are positioned as the authority on the topic, I mean you literally wrote a book about it!

If you decide to write a guide (highly suggested), I would follow a template like the one Joe Polish suggested to me.

**Below is the list of objectives that are covered in our guide.**

1. How to spot three functional medicine practice red flags

2. Six costly misconceptions about functional medicine

3. Which approach to functional medicine works best

4. Five painful mistakes to avoid when choosing a practice

5. The importance of value and price

6. Why you deserve abundant health

7. A 100 percent no-pressure guarantee

8. 4 steps to better energy, health, and vitality

To download a copy of my consumer guide, go to www.perfectpracticebook.com.

# FACEBOOK GROUP WITH WEEKLY Q&A

Another effective tool for enhancing your client experience is having a Facebook community group.

This group can consist of people from your mailing list, people who are active patients, and people who are prospective patients that want to learn more about what you do.

Remember, this group does not cost you anything, and it can benefit you if you have a lot of valuable content and information to share. It can influence a person's decision when they want to move forward and work with your practice because of the amount of value, knowledge, and wisdom that you have shared.

My wife and I do a Facebook LIVE Q&A every week, so my community can ask me whatever questions they want, whether they are patients or not. This allows me to engage and keep my ear to the ground.

It provides me with an understanding of what types of questions are coming in so I can be more effective at marketing. I can answer these questions in videos and content that we share.

Patients love the support, they enjoy the group, and it allows us to retain top-of-mind awareness with these individuals.

Members of the community love posting their questions and tuning in to hear the answer.

## Social Surveys

What's worse than creating a product or service that no one wants?

After all that time, effort, late nights, stress, anxiety, and investment – what a bust!

We've all done it!

One day I got some amazing insight into creating services that people actually want (and pay for).

I create lots a free content for my tribe, because that's what people who care about others do, right?

I get a huge rush when people resonate with my content, because it means I'm delivering value to my community.

The more value you deliver into the world, the more your efforts are rewarded with karmic currency (see later chapter on this). Not everything you do has to deliver a payday, but everything you do does have to deliver value to your audience.

By using social media to ask your audience questions, you can create highly engaging and deeply meaningful content for your audience.

If you ever want validation that you have a good idea on your hands, ask your people!

If you have a topic that you are interested in sharing more information on, just ask!

Hint: You always want validation.

Here's a great example. I recently interviewed a very special guest named Anthony Suau. He is filming a documentary called *Organic Rising*. In this documentary, he exposes the organic movement and helps people make sense of this important topic.

Check out my post on the next page.

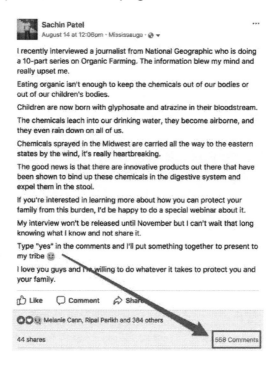

This post generated over 500 comments! Guess what webinar I'm doing next?

A simple question led to tremendous amounts of engagement and affirmation that this endeavor is worth my time. If 500 people took the time to type in yes, the odds are that that over 3,000 people are interested in the topic as a conservative estimate.

By knowing that my audience is going to love my content, I can create the information from an abundance mindset instead of a scarcity mindset. I'm not devoting any energy to wondering if people will value my work.

## Surveying Your Patients

There are several opportune times to survey your patients. Remember, surveys help you improve your services and improve the user experience. If you demonstrate to your patients that they have a say in your practice, they will help you grow it.

Why? Because they have now become part of a movement they believe in.

We survey our patients immediately after their first appointment and ask them a very important question,

---

## *"What would make this program worth your investment?"*

---

This is the most important question for you to ask every single patient. If you cannot solve this problem for them, they will never see value in your services, no matter how ideal their labs look. Remember, this whole process is for and about them, not you!

Be sure to write down any suggestions that the patient has.

We remind the patient that they will also get an email from us (automatically) with a survey for them to fill out.

In the email, we will ask what they liked about their experience and what we could have done better.

Hint: This feedback serves as a testimonial for your practice and a chance to acknowledge your team.

After each appointment, you can subtly survey your patients about how they are enjoying their experience and ask them how it can be optimized.

Take notes when they speak, and implement the changes ASAP. Once the changes have been made, kindly email the patient to let them know you appreciate the insight and that you would like to offer them a $25 credit on their next purchase at your office.

We've actually had gift cards made that we ship to the patient as our way of saying thank you. They love the acknowledgment and it reinforces this important behavior.

About three months into their program, patients will automatically receive an online survey for them to fill out (and redeem a $25 gift card). This survey is very important to acknowledge and address areas of improvement swiftly. If a patient is voicing an issue, others are probably not, so please take any suggestions seriously and, if important enough, email your patients to let them know of the improvements you've made.

Who knows? It could be the one thing keeping them from referring all their friends.

# How Can I Repurpose Content?

Creating content can seem like a daunting task unless you have a plan of action. It is important you have a strategy going into your content creation, so you can repurpose it as much as possible.

The most repurposeable content is a video. A video can be transcribed into text, and that text can be turned into a blog post, an email, or an article in a newsletter.

That same video can be uploaded to your website, YouTube, Vimeo, and Facebook. Video has the highest appeal, because it is easy for people to consume.

In fact, it is predicted that in the next few years Facebook will primarily become a video platform.

If you do not like the idea of a video or going on video makes you nervous, audio recordings are the next best thing.

You can use software like Camtasia to record whatever is on your screen and layer your voice over it. It would be more like a slideshow presentation instead of a live video of yourself.

You can also have a slideshow playing while you are presenting the information. This would be a way of getting your voice out there, for people being able to hear your passion, and for you to create video content that can be shared on various platforms. You cannot share a blog article on YouTube, but you can share a video slideshow that you create with the same content.

In this digital era, there are plenty of ways you can repurpose your content and make it extremely valuable to people by making it easy to consume.

If you are delivering webinars or if you are giving online presentations or talks, it might be of great value for you to transcribe your content and make it available as a download for people.

One of my strong recommendations is that you do Facebook LIVE events. Facebook is moving to a video platform, and these live videos have a lot of appeal.

Facebook LIVE events can be downloaded and then uploaded to YouTube. They can also be embedded on your website.

## EDUCATIONAL WORKSHOPS

One of the strategies we have found to be extremely effective is LIVE workshops and webinars. We promote our workshops through targeted Facebook ads, which then invite people to come to a free workshop or a free webinar.

During these presentations, we provide an outstanding level of education and wisdom. If information was going to save people, then guess what? They would not need you. There is plenty of information already online.

---

## Offer wisdom, rather than information

---

When people come to our live workshops, our goal is to try to create a unique experience for them: to help them feel heard, to help them ask the right questions, and to help them feel like there is hope and a solution in place.

The closer you can get to your client, (nose to nose, toes to toes) the more likely you are to get that person into your office. However, that should not be your primary objective. Your goal is to plant a seed that may sprout at any time in the future or to educate someone enough about your message that they tell others about how awesome you are.

Depending on where someone is on their journey, they may not be ready to become a patient just yet. This is likely in your best interest as well.

If people don't jump all over your compelling offer at the end, it's okay! The main question is, Will they consume future content?

Workshops are by far the most effective way for you to develop a life skill – public speaking. They are also a public platform for you to education en masse. You can educate anywhere from 10 to 50 people, even hundreds of people, in a webinar if you want to. This means you are leveraging your time more efficiently and effectively as well.

As a more advanced strategy, you can even share your webinars and live events on Facebook LIVE. Some of our events have reached thousands of people outside of the presentation room and have generated new leads and patients for us.

If you want to get strategic about this process, you can even offer a PDF download of the slideshow when people on Facebook opt in with their email address.

An even more advanced strategy can be to have people enter a key phrase in the live stream feed and have a Messenger bot segment them and send them the PDF download of the slides. This enables you to retarget these people in the future with other content.

## Taking Action After a Workshop

At the end of your workshop, you'll want to get the right people to commit to an appointment. When they come in for that appointment, you want to make sure that they are feeling heard and listened to.

The workshop is your platform to show people how passionate you are and to get people to move to a decision. That decision might be to wait until they have more information or until all their questions are answered.

People who come to a workshop are going be your warmest leads. These people have taken a tremendous amount of time out of their schedule to show up that day, and they are clearly interested in what you have to offer.

Someone who comes to a workshop is there because they are looking for help, not a free meal (because there isn't one).

When someone comes to a workshop and does not sign up for an initial consultation, you still have an opportunity to follow up with these individuals.

This could be through a series of emails that are sent as a follow-up. It could also be simply calling these individuals to see how you can support them in their journey.

A simple follow-up script might sound like this: "Hi, Mrs. Jones. I just wanted to say thank you for coming to our workshop this past weekend.

"I noticed that you filled out XYZ on your survey. We just want to make sure that you got the tools and resources that you needed out of the workshop to address these issues.

"If there is anything that we can do to help you, please let us know.

"I also wanted to let you know that you are always welcome to a future event, and if you found the information helpful, we would encourage you to share it with a friend.

"I also wanted to add you to our online Facebook community. Is that okay with you?"

Chances are this will spark a meaningful conversation and enable you to offer a discovery session at some point in the future or to get them to think of a friend that can benefit from your services.

During this call, do not try to sell them anything, but to serve them instead. Come from a place of service; this can have a profound impact on the perception of that individual.

Because this person is on a lifelong journey, you have a lifetime to get them back into your office. Just add value to their lives.

Get people to know who you are, what you represent, what you stand for, and then make sure you have an adequate follow-up with these individuals.

It might be three years from now that they come back in, or they may never come in at all, but having good relationships with these warm leads can generate many referrals and future business for you.

Be sure that you put each person into an automated sequence to further their education and escalation through your signature series.

The more you can connect with these individuals the better your odds of doing future business with them or their circle of influence.

## STRATEGIES FOR RECEIVING REFERRALS

Referrals are how we grow our business in the long run. We want to make sure we have a good solid business that people are happy to refer to.

People do business with those they know, like, and trust. Patients refer others to you if they love you, because they are attaching their name and reputation to your service.

---

## *People refer based on experience first, and results second*

---

One challenge we have when we are just starting our business is that we haven't had a chance to prove ourselves. It's going to take some time and work, possibly a year or two, to have a referral-based practice.

When patients utilize your services, they may not even know that you are accepting new patients. As hard as it may seem, you have to be willing to ask for referrals.

It can be helpful to inquire at the initial consult if the patient has someone else in mind. It's not always a good idea to ask for a referral right away, but you can ask them if they have someone who can be an accountability partner or if someone they care about can benefit from this process.
Remind them that the best way for them to learn this information is to share it with other people. We become better at what we are doing when we teach someone else what we are doing.

This is a great way for the patient to pay it forward, and if their partner hits a stumbling block, they will be much more likely to turn to your practice for assistance.

When you hold workshops or webinars, suggest to your audience to think of others who may benefit from your information.

You can also host patient appreciation or gratitude evenings and have your patients invite one to two friends they feel might benefit from this information.

Make sure your clients feel loved, appreciated, and acknowledged. Be sure that they leave every appointment with some sort of personal touch. It can be a simple email that you send at the end of the day thanking them for coming in. It's not always about the referral; it's about providing great service. A referral will be a natural byproduct of that.

Do good work, prove yourself, and make your patients feel loved.

## I'M A DOCTOR NOT A SALESPERSON

This is probably one of the most common concerns that come up when I coach practitioners.

First of all, it is important to note that you are a practitioner and educator, not a salesperson.

Health is not for sale, so there's no way that you can sell health. Health is something that must be earned, and this is why your marketing and indoctrination are extremely critical.

---

*If health was for sale,*
*no one could afford it*

---

We choose to do education-based marketing. When you do education-based marketing, you build trust with your clients and community. Our education is aligned with our core value to teach people how to stay out of our office. It might seem counterintuitive, but it works because it builds trust.

Education-based marketing allows people to make their own decision based on new information being presented to them.

"People don't change their mind, they make new decisions with new information" – Zig Ziglar

# ESSENTIAL TECHNOLOGY

# The Essential Digital Tools

There are several essential tools to help your practice in the online, education, and marketing space. Keep in mind that digital tools are constantly evolving, and new ones are being released all the time.

If you do not use the specific tools I recommend, find similar tools that can help you accomplish the same tasks. Just remember, it's better to start with what you need to eliminate hurdles in your growth later.

You'll want tools to capture and nurture leads, host your content, provide easy communication, and process payments.

These software services will make your life so much easier and enable you to reach millions of people if your heart desires. The nice thing about many of these tools is that they scale with your practice. This means that costs are contained as your practice grows.

**The five essential tools that I suggest are.**

1. Active Campaign
2. Click Funnels
3. Zoom
4. Kajabi
5. Stripe

With these five services 90 percent of your online needs will be met.

## Active Campaign

Active Campaign is customer relationship management software. This is where your leads are handled. You should manage your prospective clients here, as well as your existing patients.

Active Campaign allows you to track open rates and click rates, and to score your audience based on their levels of engagement. The more engaged someone is with your content, the more appropriate it would be for your team to reach out to them or send them very specific emails or content.

## Click Funnels

Click Funnels is an amazing software that allows you to build custom landing pages and funnels for your sales process. It's a very easy software to use and it integrates very nicely with Active Campaign.

## Zoom

Another important program that you should have is called Zoom. Zoom is an online alternative to Skype, and I find it much easier to use. It is great for interviews, and you can also host webinars that stream directly to Facebook LIVE or YouTube LIVE.

Zoom is HIPAA compliant, so you can interview your patients on it as well. It is easy to record to your computer or to the cloud. Zoom is the go-to platform for your video needs.

## Kajabi

Online courses are a great way to curate your knowledge and expertise. Kajabi provides you with a robust platform to create courses.

The software is designed by Brandon Burchard and is very easy to use. It is a little on the pricey side, but the point of your course is to sell it and recover your investment.

## Stripe

If you are taking online payments, you will want an online payment processor that is easy to use and that syncs very easily with your Click Funnel, Active Campaign, and Kajabi account.

The service we use is called Stripe. Stripe is an online payment processor that syncs very easily and easy for developers to work with.

Running the practice of the future means that you'll want to have the right tools to help you scale your message and automate your influence. These tools are an excellent place to start.

You can find a complete list of apps when you register at www.perfectpracticebook.com.

# THE CHARACTERISTICS OF A GREAT WEBSITE

One of the most important tools you have is your online business card: your website. Your website might be one of the first things that people see when searching for the solution you are offering.

Discussing the ins and outs of a website requires a lengthier discussion, but the next few pages should get you started.

Your website should be easy to follow and laid out well on every platform. Be sure you test your website on multiple different operating systems and browsers before you give your developer the final thumbs up.

Your website should be easy on the eyes. Keep in mind that most people will visit your website from their mobile phones, so be sure the mobile experience of your website is very user-friendly.

Your website should be representative of your brand feel. Be sure to use images that portray the desired outcome of your patients instead of pain.

Every page on your site should be designed to capture a contact's email address with a compelling call to action and "ethical bribe" in return.

According to Facebook marketer Nicholas Kusmich, be sure to have a desirable and easy-to-consume lead magnet on your website, such as a PDF download that gives your client a quick win!

A good example could be a morning routine guide or a sleep guide to help with better healing energy. A short PDF that is nicely done will capture way more leads than a sales call. Although they will be required later in the onboarding process, it's best to lead with a PDF download and escalate people through your educational funnels.

What's a brand-aligned download that you can offer people to get them started on their journey with your company?

The image below is a quick reference for you to correctly position your offering on your website.

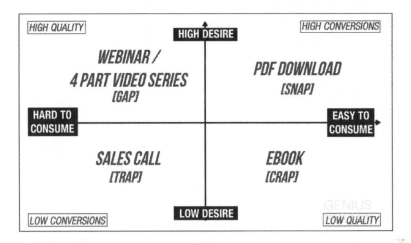

I highly recommend you work with a website developer who is familiar with the functional medicine space. This is important for keeping your brand integrity and messaging intact.

An experienced web developer will have a keen eye for detail but also be familiar with your messaging and ensure you get the best product possible.

# FACEBOOK PIXELS

Pixels are a fancy little digital tracker that can be embedded into the code of any page on your website. Pixels can track and then follow users after they have engaged with your content.

At some point, you've probably gone to Amazon and changed your mind about a purchase and then abandoned your shopping cart.

Shortly afterward you probably noticed ads from Amazon and the exact product you were searching for magically start appearing everywhere on the internet. This is known as retargeting and is powered by pixels.

When installed and set up properly, pixels can trigger a variety of predetermined events. For example, if you're driving traffic to a blog article and someone clicks on the link to go to your website, it might make sense to retarget that person with more similar content on your website or promote an upcoming webinar that you're hosting.

Different pixels can be installed on different pages of your website and at various stages in your cart or online funnels. They really are a powerful tool that can help you attract and escalate new leads for pennies on the dollar!

## SHARING CASE STUDIES

Your website should have case studies and testimonials. Case studies are a very powerful way of demonstrating how you help patients, not just what you have done but how you have actually helped them.

Because functional medicine is a relatively new concept to most people, they often do not even realize what they do not know.

Remember the first time you saw a functional lab test and how excited you were?

Prospects have probably never seen one before, and you can create the same level of excitement for them, helping them know that they may have finally found answers.

We share case studies in short, three- to eight-minute videos, and we post these as often as possible. We walk viewers through the presentation of the patient, what their chief complaint and pain points were, what things their discomfort or issues were preventing them from doing, what they had done previously, what we uncovered through their history that was missed, what lab testing we ordered, what protocol we put them on, and what the outcomes were.

We try to connect with the viewer as best we can by including details that might build that relationship. We have had several new patient consults result from sharing these case studies online, because readers felt like we were speaking to them.

Testimonials are also great, but they do not showcase how in-depth your work is or what was actually done to produce the outcomes. Chances are every single person they saw before you probably also had testimonials of how great their services were on their website.

Case studies can dive deeper into the outcome you can produce for people and how you are going to produce it. They highlight how you are going to do things differently than what they have tried before.

Be sure to check the laws where you practice concerning sharing case studies on your website or social media. In some places even removing the name is not enough.

To see examples of case studies, visit our website at www.becomeproof.com

## ONLINE QUIZZES

Another effective online tool is a quiz. A quiz is a way to qualify patients based on their need and on their readiness. Having a quiz easily accessible in your website menu is a great way to engage people and capture leads, as well as move people through your automation.

We quiz every patient before having them schedule a free phone consultation. This gives us insights into their pain points and helps us understand a little bit more about what they are going through.

When we speak to their pain points and symptoms, prospects feel heard for the first time. Sometimes they even forget what they told you in the quiz, making you seem like a psychic during the call!

Keep your quiz short but meaningful, and be sure to follow up with each lead. Someone who fills out a quiz is looking for answers.

Keep in mind that they may not be ready to instantly become a patient, but you can at least point them to the right resources to help them find some answers on your website.

Check out our online quiz here: http://bit.ly/LPIQuiz

## Sharing Your Message through Videos

I highly encourage having video content on your website. Video content can include videos of yourself sharing information or interviews. They build a much deeper bond and relationship with you and your prospective clients.

You will feel extremely valued when your patients come see you, because you have built up this relationship with them through the videos on your website.

Keep your videos informative, demonstrate your wisdom, and give people valuable tips so that they can take action and reap some sort of benefit.

Video is the richest content. A video can birth a blog article, it can increase search ranking in Google, and it can be embedded in multiple places (Facebook, YouTube, Vimeo, etc.).

Videos on your website should appear thoughtful but don't have to be super professionally done. Most smartphones these days, combined with good lighting and a tripod, are all you need. Remember that content is king, so be sure you have clear audio to catch the information.

The more you overthink the process, the less likely you are to do it. I have found that my most watched videos are ones that I do on the fly, from my car, from my balcony, or when I'm out and about. I guess they are just more relatable at the end of the day.

# THE BENEFITS OF AN AUTORESPONDER?

One of the most important assets your business will ever grow is your email list. Your email list is critical, because it keeps your clients on your platform. It is great to have a ton of Instagram and Facebook followers, but guess who owns those contacts?

This means you have to contact them through Facebook's platform. That is not always the most efficient way to get in front of your audience. It is also difficult to know who your audience is and how engaged they are in your content unless you have some statistics.

For example, when someone reads your post on Facebook, there is no way for you to know they read that post. In fact, even if someone likes the post they may not have read the whole thing or fully immersed themselves in the content.

Collecting people's email addresses is very important, because you can then send them information through your customer relationship management (CRM) software like Active Campaign.

By having people enter into specific opt-ins that are geared towards their interests, you are able to segment your list. This means you can have different landing pages for different topics and nurture your list accordingly. This way people who want information on one specific condition only get information, promotion, and invites to events associated with that particular interest.

## KNOWING YOUR AUDIENCE

Another reason to build a list is that through your CRM software you are able to identify who is more engaged with your content, who is opening your emails, who is clicking on your links, and how many emails someone has been engaged with before they call your office to make an appointment.

There are many little bits of information that allow you to better understand your customer. If I am going to get a call from a prospective patient, or even from a practitioner, I can pull up their account in my CRM software, pinpoint their name and email address, and look at their engagement history.

By looking at the links they have clicked on, the emails they have opened, and the amount of engagement they have had with our content, it helps me better understand where they are in their journey.

If a patient or a practitioner is just starting out and engaging with our content, it is important for me to share information that will be helpful for that part of their journey.

If this person has been engaged in my content for a couple of years now, it is probably time to move them towards a buying decision if that is the next right step for them. The only way to know this information is by having a CRM like Active Campaign.

I recently consulted with a colleague of mine. He's been on several radio shows and TV shows in his hometown, and because of that he has gained a tremendous amount of recognition. He has been doing this for several years, so I asked him a simple question, "How big is your email list?" He replied, "What email list?"

All this time he has missed the opportunity to capture tens of thousands of emails and provide so much service, value, and engagement with these individuals.

He never had a compelling offer to make them, and he did not have a landing page to drive traffic to or a CRM to capture the

106

information. He could have even retargeted those people on Facebook or through Google Ads. Needless to say, a huge opportunity was missed!

Your CRM is a critical tool to grow your brand, improve your customer experience, and deliver high-quality content and value at the right time to your audience.

This topic deserves an entire book to itself, but in the meantime, start by getting a simple account set up with Active Campaign to start capturing and nurturing your leads.

# I'M NOT TECH SAVVY!

As a clinician who is navigating a new paradigm of healthcare, it might not be in your best interest to try to also become a digital technician.

My recommendation is for you to learn enough about a particular platform to know when you're getting ripped off and when someone is providing you with value.

In my mentorship, I show practitioners step-by-step how to get specific things done. This includes setting up a landing page, setting up an automation, and setting up a series of educational emails.

Some of these steps can be extremely easy. Other things, like custom integrations and APIs, can be a lot more confusing. It might be more effective from an emotional standpoint, and from a cost standpoint, to hire a professional to do those things.

One of my recommendations is to hire people that others in your industry have used and can vet. It is much easier to hire someone who understands what your business is about, because they have worked with someone in your industry.

It is also reassuring that someone you trust has used this vendor. When a colleague uses a vendor, a lot of the heavy lifting and explaining has been done for you. This will minimize the amount of back and forth that will take place.

You probably would not expect a web developer to try to become a functional medical practitioner, so you should not expect a functional medical practitioner to become a web developer. Work with people who are known in the industry to provide good work and leverage a good referral.

Unless you're going to get paid to help others develop digital content at some point in the future, it's best to hire the right help to get the work done!

You've already got enough on your plate; you don't need to worry about learning a whole new skill set. The nice thing about your digital architecture is that once it's set up, you're good to go!

Anything that slows you down slows down the process of getting your message in front of thousands of people, so the sooner you can get the help you need to set up your systems, the better!

For a list of trusted providers visit, www.perfectpracticebook.com.

# MONEY MINDSET

## Karmic Currency

Today, more than ever, it's possible for you to help someone and deliver tremendous value, even if they never use your paid services.

This is what I call karmic currency. Karmic currency means if you do something good for someone, even if they don't pay you, there will be positive dividends resulting from your efforts. This is a universal law.

It is important we use more than one metric to measure our success in life and business. In the sales world, success is measured only by conversions and income. It's strictly a numbers game for some people; I encourage you not to fall into the trap.

In the functional medicine world and in the world of healing, our mantra is, "Does our client get better as a result of interacting and engaging with us?"

A client can enjoy better health by coming to your workshop and making some of the changes that you discussed. This can be done without coming into your office.

A client can get better by simply filling out your intake form, sitting down with you and discussing it for an hour, and making changes that you recommended.

Of course, a client can also get better if they work with you over a period of time.

All three of the above scenarios produce the same healing energy and a corresponding karmic result. In one scenario, you didn't get paid anything. In the second scenario, you got paid a little. In the third scenario, you got paid for the services that you offered that person.

Karmic currency is much more valuable than money in your bank account for a variety of reasons. This type of currency results in amazing opportunities and circumstances presenting themselves to you or your business.

When you do good work with the right intention to serve others, amazing people and situations start showing up in your life. Circumstances that no amount of money can buy will start presenting themselves in your life.

The redemption of karmic currency requires both awareness and gratitude combined with a genuine desire to give instead of take.

---

## *Karmic currency is the most important type of wealth to build*

---

One thing I've learned over the years that has served me tremendously is to give with no expectations. When we set expectations, we set ourselves up for disappointment and a reward that is based on our limiting beliefs. The universe might have a bigger plan for us!

# DO YOUR CLIENTS THINK YOU'RE EXPENSIVE?

If a patient is working with you, they should never feel like they are paying too much. The right client who has the right level of education about your process, who has enough social proof, who trusts you and likes you, or who was referred to you should always happily pay your fees.

The right client will take that fee and turn it into far more value than what they are actually paying you.

If someone thinks that your services are expensive, guess what they are telling others.

If you ever hear your patients saying, "I want to refer my friend but I don't think she can afford it," the problem lies in the fact that not enough value has been created for the price your client is paying.

**This is destroying your referrals!**

My suggestion would be to offer that patient's referral a free phone call to assess if they are a good fit or a chance to point them to the free resources they need to move forward in their journey. This is where your free tools can really serve those in need and escalate them appropriately through your signature series.

Chances are your patient doesn't have the full story of what challenges the prospect is facing. People don't tell their friends everything about their health; most people downplay the issue.

## GIVERS GAIN

This is the universal law of exchange. It is very important that you understand this and read this chapter with an open heart and an open mind.

Your healthcare business exists to solve your client's healthcare issues first, not to solve your personal financial issues. When you solve other people's problems, rest assured that your problems will be solved.

As a functional medicine practitioner, chances are you are not doing this for the Ferrari or the 8,000 square foot home. While both of those things are completely acceptable goals, they should not be the primary focus of why you do business.

---

*The amount of money you make is directly proportional to the value you deliver into the marketplace*

---

We should deliver ten times more value than what people pay us. If you deliver tens of millions of dollars of value into the marketplace, you have to be okay with receiving millions of dollars in return.

Realize that the other 90 percent is paid through karmic currency – which creates outcomes and circumstances that money can't buy!

## THE ENERGY EXCHANGE

If you want to make a lot of money, there are easier ways you can do it besides going into functional medicine.

Some people will tell you love of money is the root of all evil. I believe money is the fruit of all good. Money can be used to do great things, and money can be used to do horrible things.

---

## *Money is stored energy*

---

You can pay someone money to move a few boxes for you, or you can pay a team member to create a landing page for you, and they release the energy stored in that money and create work in exchange for more stored energy (money).

Keep in mind that your knowledge and experience are also stored energy waiting to change form.

Energy cannot be created or destroyed; it can only change forms. I truly believe that when there is a mismatch between the value delivered and the amount of money exchanged, there is very little flow in that direction.

This means if you are undercharging, do not expect the universe to reward you. If you are overcharging, do not expect the universe to reward you either.

## MONEY IS RARELY THE MAIN ISSUE

You might say, "No one can afford my services." Or "People who are really ill cannot afford my services." One thing for you to keep in mind is that the true problem is very rarely money. Your clients are driving to your offices in cars that cost 10–20 times more than what your case fees are, and they are living in homes that are 100 to 200 times your case fees.

Money is not the main issue; it is the perception that is the main issue. If a client has the wrong perception of you, if they do not trust you, or if they feel like you are charging too much, they probably have not been properly qualified to truly understand what you have to offer them.

Money is not a great qualifier for functional medicine patients; value perception and compliance are much better qualifiers.

A great patient is someone who values your services more than they value digits in on a computer screen.

You want to work with people who truly value what you bring to the table and understand the thousands of hours of training that you have done to be able to deliver your services.

Grateful clients will honor the fact that you are running a business, and that you need to stay in business to serve your community.

## Who Does the Money Serve Best?

One concept that might be difficult for some people to wrap their heads around, but that has helped me tremendously, is that

---

*if you don't need the money right now, it doesn't matter whose bank account that money is in*

---

Once the value exchanges hands, the money will change bank accounts.

If the money your prospect has serves them better in their own bank account, let them keep their money. Do not create a problem that you cannot fix!

If that money serves them better by paying you for your services and you can deliver way more value than what that money is worth in their bank account, then it's your obligation to do business with this individual, and you should both feel good about it.

Your ideal patients should feel good about the value they are receiving in exchange for the money they are paying. As a general rule of thumb, ask your patient, "what would make this program worth 10 times more than what you pay us?" Then listen carefully and take notes!

## BEING PAID INDIRECTLY

If you do not need the money right now, do not get hung up on the fact that people are asking you for free information and advice.

The reason people ask you for advice is because they trust you. It is very easy for people to go on their phones, jump on Google, and ask a question.

However, the reason they ask you is because they trust you. I gladly answer their questions and continue to build trust. Eventually the energy will exchange.

The funny thing about money is that the people you deliver the most value to are not always the ones who pay you. Remember that money is energy, and energy comes in many forms.

This could be in the form of good relationships, it could be in the form of serendipity, it could be in the form of opportunity, it could be in the form of a good night's sleep or in the form of other amazing things.

This is why gratitude and mindfulness are so important. They help us recognize the many forms in which we are paid.

*Energy can take on many forms, and money just happens to be one of them.*

*If we look at the pie of life, money is the smallest sliver of that pie.*

*Make sure you are practicing gratitude and awareness, and that you are paying attention to all the amazing things that are happening in your life as a result of your go-giver attitude.*

*Do not get overly hung up on your bank account, because you will miss the big picture.*

## REFUNDS AND RELATIONSHIPS

There will be times when patients come into your life who don't see value in the care that you offer.

Perhaps it is because they are not willing to do the work, or they underestimated the changes that needed to take place.

My suggestion to you is to refund the money to these individuals as quickly and as swiftly as possible.

These people essentially act like boulders in your river. They are never going to refer anyone to you. As long as you have their money, they will probably talk negatively about you. They are costing you way more money than you having their money is providing value for you.

I would highly encourage that you periodically survey your patients, especially those that are unresponsive to your emails, and promptly issue a refund to them for unused services. People who do not see value in your work or who are not committed to doing the work will never send you patients, especially patients that will take action.

After working with thousands of people, I've only had to issue a refund a few times. To be perfectly honest, it felt amazing to release this dark energy from my bank account.

Since like attracts like, get rid of this negative energy from your space, and make room for more positive energy from people who value your efforts.

## You're Not A Charity!

You might say, "What about those people that can't afford our services? What can we do to help them?"

If someone can't afford your services, chances are you won't be able to do your job. The worst thing that you can do is lower your fees and take someone's money who cannot fully follow through with your recommendations.

You would never sell someone who is broke a BMW, because that person will never be able to take advantage of the performance that that car has to offer if they are not putting in premium fuel and taking the best care of the car. Over time the car will become a huge burden.

Have you ever seen those reality shows where they help someone rebuild a home and then the family cannot afford the taxes on the home?

You have to decide what type of service you want to deliver. Do you want to be the best, or do you want to be a commodity and try to be the cheapest?

---

*"You have got to see my functional medicine doc, they're the cheapest," said no one, ever!*

---

You should only work with clients who can truly afford your care. You will be doing these people a huge disservice otherwise.

If you're trying to save your patients money, get them healthy. At the end of the day, saving patients a couple of thousand dollars is really not going to have a big impact on their life. It is a very minuscule amount in the grand scheme of things.

If you're trying to save patients a few hundred bucks by compromising the possibility of saving them tens of thousands and living ten years longer, then you are committing a crime, in my opinion.

Your job isn't to save people money, because – let's face it – you're going to help people do the most expensive thing possible: live longer!

## CHARGING BASED ON VALUE

The formality of charging people is just that. It is a formality in exchange for the value that you are delivering. You should feel happy and proud that you have the ability to transform patients' lives and that whatever they pay you is going to multiply 10 times in terms of value.

A very busy functional medicine practice will enroll 30 to 50 new patients a month, depending on the size of your city or town. That is a drop in the bucket compared to the number of people that are out there.

Through effective marketing, relationship building and the right indoctrination, you will be able to attract those 30 to 50 new clients without any problems.

Poor money mindset is the number one thing holding practitioners back, and it is completely understandable based on what practitioners go through.

Insurance companies have been beating us down, paying us less and less every year. Patients feel entitled to get the cheapest services possible, and they expect doctors to give away their services for free or for little to no cost.

Most people do not realize the amount of work that goes into running a business and offering healthcare services. Most people do not realize how draining it can be for practitioners.

Prospects may not always realize that to get the best service possible, they have got to be willing to pay for it.

They have to be able to trust that you are not ripping them off and that you are providing tremendous value for the price they are paying. I would never take a patient that felt like my services were expensive, because that means they do not see the value in the care I am providing.

I only take patients that see tremendous value in my services, who do not question my fees, and who are excited to engage in my care. I suggest that you do the same.

## Your Services Are Priceless

The majority of the work you and your patient do will not be in your face-to-face encounters.

It's important to note that the value of your services is determined by the client and the level of action that they take when they leave your office.

The value of your services is $0 if the client takes no action or does not take your care seriously. It is critical you have the right education and steps in place to attract your ideal client into your office.

---

*You want someone coming to you because you are the best, not because you are the cheapest*

---

Your price will vary based on a few variables.

First, it is important to get a clear understanding of what you are offering your client. Is your offer only the one-on-one time that you are spending, or is there more to it? Are you offering group classes? Are you offering email access to you? Are you offering online support through a Facebook group or live Q&A? Are you offering additional resources such as an online course?

These are all critical questions to ask and effort for you to value. If you do not value these things, certainly your patients will not.

Many patients come from a paradigm where they are simply paying for a procedure code. They are going in, getting a service, and leaving. Then the service and process end.

Typically, with functional and lifestyle medicine, the service begins when the patient leaves your office because now they are going to be able to act on the steps that you have laid out for them.

The value of what you offer also extends into their immediate network of family and friends who may also benefit from the knowledge they are receiving from you for generations to come.

When paired with a motivated and committed patient, your services are truly priceless.

Let that sink in for a moment!

## BE CONFIDENT IN WHAT YOUR TIME IS WORTH

Your confidence ties into what you will charge. Many practitioners have a scarcity mindset, and they are afraid of charging what their time is actually worth, driven by a fear of failure. Your fear of failure served you in school, but it's not going to serve you in business.

---

## *People who fear failure aim low*

---

Sometimes this lack of confidence can arise from poor subconscious programming that you had nothing to do with.

When you fear failure, you undercharge and get overworked.

Initially, this might seem noble, but you cannot do business if you are not in business.

You cannot help people if your practice no longer exists and you are burnt out as a practitioner.

The best thing that you can do to help people who can't afford your services is offer free touch points such as Facebook groups, an email newsletter, videos on social media, and an automated responder sequence that allows people to take care of some of the most fundamental changes that they can make. There are many ways we can help people for free.

Use the ideas suggested in this book to create programs to serve your community at any level and create enough value for your time and wisdom that people gladly pay you your fees because they are fair and you deliver exceptional value.

It's important to note that good fortune only comes to those that pay it forward; money is an energy that likes to flow. Think of it as a battery.

What fun is a battery if it never gets used? The battery wants to put a smile on a child's face when it's put into a toy. It doesn't want to sit in your sock drawer for ten years and lose its charge.

Let the energy flow be learning how to pay it forward to causes and efforts you believe in.

## PAY IT FORWARD

Remember to always pay it forward to those that are in true need. One of the ways that you can do that is to pick a local organization or charity in your community that you and your team believe in.

You can sponsor this organization and contribute a portion of your proceeds every year to their fund. It is a great way for your patients to know you're paying it forward.

They will know their money is going towards a good cause, and not just for you to buy that fancy car or that lavish home. When we start every financial planning session, we do not start with how much we want to make; we start with how much we want to give and reverse engineer the solution from there.

Thanks to the concepts in this book and our supportive community, we've been able to donate tens of thousands of dollars to help build a hospital in Butebi, Uganda, and support an entire village's healthcare needs.

# 10 WAYS TO PAY IT FORWARD

## 1. Quick tips on Facebook

Allow people to take immediate action and see immediate wins. You want people to win without having to do too much. If they have to go through a complicated process to get something in return, you might not see them again. Give them a quick win, and be consistent. You want to be consistently delivering information that helps people. If you are consistent, you will stand out in your community, because no one else is doing it.

## 2. Facebook groups

We have a Facebook group that is open to patients and prospective patients. It is open to anyone who wants to join. We share tips and recipes every day. You can join here www.lpicommunity.com

## 3. Volunteer somewhere

Put that energy out there! Connect with a cause you believe in and involve your tribe and your patients as much as you can. People love helping others; it's human nature.

## 4. Donate

Donate financially to causes that you believe in. I often involve my community if I am making a contribution, so they can be involved. People love donating if they know the money is doing good work.

## 5. Prepare things people can download

Offer e-books, guides, cookbooks, or checklists that people can download for free. That is an easy win for them and something they can benefit from.

## 6. In-office workshops

Nurture your patients. Try to deliver as much value to your existing clients as you can by offering workshops. Allow them to bring friends or family members. Often this can lead to new referrals, and it gives a great deal of value to the people who attend.

## 7. Forever gratitude journals

In our office, we give out gratitude journal called The Five-Minute Journal to every patient. Patients write in them every morning and every evening. As a result of that, they hopefully think about us when they are writing in them. They are practicing gratitude, and gratitude has been shown to be very beneficial for healing. Every time they bring back a completed journal to show us, we give them another one for free, for life!

## 8. Become a better receiver

If you become a better receiver, you can become a better giver. The cycle has to be fulfilled. The better you are at receiving, the more good you can do for others. If I'm not good at receiving money or good energy, that energy will not find its way to me for me to give it to other people.

## 9.Value-driven webinars

Set up a webinar where you are not trying to sell anything. Offer a webinar to collectively solve a problem or to offer valuable information for those attending. You don't always have to have a pitch. The relationship with your audience is the most important part of a webinar, not the pitch.

## 10. Help others get what they want

It doesn't get simpler than that, but there is a key point to make here. You can only discover what people want when you ask them what they want first.

Hint: Helping others doesn't have to always have to be in a functional medicine capacity. Think of creative ways that you can contribute to the betterment of the world around you!

# MENTORSHIP

## Should I Join a Mentorship?

The truth is, I don't know.

Mentorship has been one of the most rewarding experiences of my professional life. Mentorship has provided me with such amazing insights into myself, into my business, and into the future of both.

Mentorship provides unbiased insights and the opportunity for practitioners to share what they have learned along their journey. After coaching over one hundred practitioners, I have realized that mentorship has been one of the most rewarding professional experiences for them as well.

There are certain attributes of people who benefit from mentorship. Just like most things, mentorship is not for everyone. It takes a certain caliber of individual to benefit from a mentorship or mastermind group.

It is not just what you get out of the process, but it is also who you become through the process and how you contribute to the success of other people who are part of the same mentorship or mastermind.

I recently posed a question in my group about the attributes of someone who should join a mentorship group. Here they are:

1. People who believe in themselves: You must believe in what you bring to the table and what you have to offer the world. Without this core belief, no matter what program or process you engage in, you will never be successful.

   It begins with believing in ourselves, the ability to carry out and execute orders, and the ability to take constructive feedback and criticisms so we can aggressively expand our mission.

2. People who believe the market needs their services sooner rather than later: There is no doubt in my mind that anyone who is reading this book can accomplish the same things I have. However, I strongly doubt that you can do it in the same amount of time that you would be able to do if it wasn't through a mentorship.

   A mentorship allows you to skip all the mistakes and errors, and it allows you to avoid unnecessary hindsight that leaves you kicking yourself. The market likely needs your services now.

   The longer you take to get your program in process and your systems together, the longer your audience suffers and the more they suffer, the more likely they are to choose someone else to fulfill their immediate needs.

3. People who realize the power of community: Community is extremely important to your success. How you interact and engage with other people is very important in determining how successful you and your business will become.

   When you connect with other like-minded people who are on a similar journey, you have the collective power of their brains, experiences, and insights.

Working in a community like ours, for example, allows you to tap into several hundred years of collective experience in the exact industry your business is positioned in. The value these people bring to the table is extremely powerful.

4. People who deeply value their time: Time is our most essential and important asset. Mentorship can save you significant amounts of time, because a lot of the thinking is essentially done for you.

   A lot of the hard work and heavy lifting is done for you. Most of us may not realize this, but time is fleeting. It is not something we can ever get back. Money can be replenished, but time cannot. Mentorship can save you years of anguish and frustration.

5. People who like to time travel: The closest thing I can think of to time travel is mentorship and the wisdom you gain from other people.

   You do not have to go through the same learning journeys those people have, as long as you are open to learning from what they have to share.

   Some things we have to learn the hard way, but most things, especially strategy, we can learn quite easily from other people. By being in a mentorship group, you can accelerate past typical timelines of getting things done.

   One of the things we offer in our mentorship is marketing collateral and patient collateral. This allows you to focus on building your business, while someone else is helping you build your messaging and other aspects of your platform. While you are sleeping or while you are seeing patients, work is being done on your behalf. This is what I call time travel.

6. People who realize that one idea can change everything: People who join mentorships usually pick up on this very quickly.

   They are after are deep and valuable insights, not necessarily a line item by line item utilization of everything that a mentorship offers. It is impossible and frustrating for someone to leverage every single tool a mentorship can offer.

   What is important is to keep your eyes and ears open for the things that can be transformational for you. The value of an entire mentorship can boil down to one thing that you needed to hear at the right time, that diverted you from years of anguish, or that promoted you in the right direction so you can leverage your skillset.

   I have had conversations that have been worth several hundred thousand dollars, because of the ripple effect of that conversation and my ability to take that information and run with it. I have also had conversations that have saved me thousands of dollars. The advice from other people prevented me from going down the wrong path.

7. People who recognize that who you know is more important than what you know: I've learned over the years that building connections with people is extremely valuable.

   Knowing people who are connected with certain individuals is also extremely valuable. One of my keys to success, in accelerating to the top of the functional medicine space, is through my contacts.

   I've put in work. I've put in effort, like many of you reading this book probably have. However, what has gotten me to the top is the connections and relationships I have made along the way.

Many of you reading this book might actually be better practitioners than I am. The question is: do you have better connections than I do? By joining a mentorship, you are instantly connected to my network.

When someone is looking for a practitioner who has the same skillset, guess who I am going to prioritize when that opportunity arises? Who you know is much more important than what you know, and most people tend to focus on what they know.

8. People who are coachable: Being coachable is very important, because someone who is mentoring you or coaching you is going to see a side of you that you cannot see. They are going to see blind spots that you are completely unaware of.

    We call this unconscious incompetence. You do not even know you have a problem. No matter how nice or expensive your car is, every car has a blind spot. A mentor can help you discover what those blind spots are, but you have to be coachable to accept those blind spots and actually do something about them.

9. People who take ownership over their outcomes: You have to be willing to take complete ownership over your outcomes. When things go wrong, you take ownership. When things go right, you take ownership.

    People who take ownership over their outcomes are people who continue to grow and learn from their mistakes. They learn from their successes and their mistakes and continue to improve upon them.

10. People who realize that readiness is far greater than responsiveness: I believe success is a result of readiness, not responsiveness. When I am looking to work with someone, I want someone who is ready, not someone who is responsive to everything I say. No

matter how responsive you are, you may not necessarily be ready.

Mentorship shows you what areas in life and in business you need to be ready in, not just areas you have to respond in. Responsiveness is good, but there is still a delay time. When you are ready, things can start moving extremely quickly for you.

11. People who realize they have a higher calling: People who have a higher calling usually recognize the fact that it is going to take more than themselves to take their mission and purpose to the next level.

   It is critical you surround yourself with like-minded people and like-minded individuals, because typically your calling is much bigger than you. You are going to need a team of people supporting you.

12. People who do work that is in complete alignment with their core values: Typically, masterminds and mentorship are hand-picked and extremely curated individuals. You have to make sure whatever mentorship group you are in aligns with your core values and you operate out of your core values in every single thing that you do. When you do that, amazing things start happening for you personally and in your business: your sleep improves, your energy improves, your motivation improves, and the type of people and circumstances that show up in your life improve. This is because they are all aligned with your deepest values.

13. People who love to collaborate: In a mentorship, you have a unique ability to collaborate with individuals who are on a similar mission as you.

   Chances are somebody else has probably done the work that you are trying to do right now. Or chances are you have done the work that someone else is trying to do right now.

By collaborating with other individuals, you can improve the work of other people, and you can work as a team to optimize the work that has already been done.

14. People who invest in growth and want to raise their game most efficiently by modeling a proven method: When you belong to a mentorship group, usually the people in the group are modeling a method that works, or they are testing a method that may work.

    You can learn from their wins, you can learn from their mistakes, and you can optimize your process to suit your needs. Working in a mentorship provides a template for you to work with so you can grow as quickly as possible.

15. People who want to be held accountable: Accountability is extremely important. It is difficult to be held accountable to someone who does not really understand what you do.

    People around us, our best friends, and sometimes even our spouses may not fully understand what it is that we do. The problems that we approach these individuals with may fall on deaf ears. They may not be able to provide sound advice to us, because they do not really understand what our problem is or how to help us efficiently.

    By being part of a mentorship, you will be held accountable by other individuals who understand your problems and can provide you with extremely valuable insights and advice.

16. People who are team players: Being in a mentorship means that you are going to be playing for a team, typically a winning team.

    How much you contribute to that winning team will determine how much you get out of the entire process as well. Just like on a team, it is important you contribute to the best of your ability, ask questions, and raise awareness around certain blind spots other people might have. When you are playing on a team, you might shout out to your teammates, "Hey, watch out on your right," because that person might get blindsided if they don't.

By helping other people and realizing that other people will help you, you can have much more confidence and clarity when you are taking action.

17. People who have an abundance mindset: Typically, people who join mastermind groups and mentorships have a very strong abundance mindset.

These individuals realize that the more they give, the more they get. They are happy to contribute. They realize that by creating something and having a hundred other eyes on it, someone can find a way to make that process better.

The most important things that have ever been accomplished were accomplished by teams of people. We did not go to the moon with just one person working on the project.

We did not go into the deepest depths of the ocean by one person working on the project. Anything important that has ever been done has been a team effort.

Each of these individuals had an abundance mindset, because they realized the more they give and contribute, the more they have to gain from the process.

18. People who want to have freedom and make an impact: By working in collaboration in a mentorship or a mastermind, you are freeing up your time

You are not replicating work that has already been done. You can have a much bigger impact this way, because if the heavy lifting is already done for you, it is not going to take you months or years to get the message out there.

You can start getting the message out there immediately and strategically, and have a much bigger impact, much sooner.

19. People who want to pay it forward: One of the best ways to learn something is not to just learn it; it is to teach it to other people. The people in a mentorship are going to be very happy to pay their knowledge, their wisdom, and their experiences forward.

   This will help you move aggressively in the right direction and have success. It is important you do the same thing. It is always important in any area of our lives to pay it forward. Sometimes we can pay it forward by knowledge, sometimes we can pay it forward through financial means, and sometimes we can pay it forward by donating our time.

   People with an abundance mindset recognize there is an infinite reservoir from which they can contribute, especially once they find their voice and combine it with their passion.

20. People who want to spend more time with their family: By being part of a mentorship and having a lot of the heavy work done for you, this frees up your time. You might spend this time researching or creating. You can spend more time doing the things you love. You can spend time with your family, pursue hobbies, or travel.

   Being in mentorships has helped me tremendously over the years. It is something I recommend to all my colleagues. Whether it is a mentorship in our program or another program that suits your needs, I would highly encourage that you take it into strong consideration.

This will allow you to get your message out there to as many people as possible, as quickly as possible, and to end the needless suffering that is currently going on.

**Here's a quick checklist of the above points, check all those that apply and add up your score at the bottom.**

- ❏ People who believe in themselves

- ❏ People who believe the market needs their services sooner, rather than later

- ❏ People who realize the power of community

- ❏ People who deeply value their time

- ❏ People who like to time travel

- ❏ People who realize that one idea can change everything

- ❏ People who realize that: who you know >>> what you know

- ❏ People who are coachable

- ❏ People who take ownership over their outcomes

- ❏ People who realize that readiness >>> responsiveness

- ❏ People who realize that they have a higher calling

- ❏ People who do work that is in complete alignment with their core values

- ❏ People who love to collaborate

- ❏ People who invest in growth and want to raise their game by modeling a proven method

- ❏ People who want to be held accountable

- ❏ People who are team players

- ❏ People who have an abundance mindset

- ❏ People who want to have freedom and make an impact

- ❏ People who pay it forward

- ❏ People who want to spend more time with their family

Total:   /20

What's your score?

If it's over 18/20, I would love to speak with you personally and see if working together is a good fit to help you build, grow, and scale your functional medicine practice.

## LET'S CONNECT

Thank you for taking the time to read this book. I hope that it has provided you with a better perspective on how you can become a pillar of hope for your community.

Your community needs to you now more than ever!

I've helped over 100 practitioners build, grow, and scale their functional medicine practices.

If you're interested in working together, you can learn more about our mentorship program and set up a call with me here: http://bit.ly/mentorwithsachin.

# ABOUT SACHIN PATEL

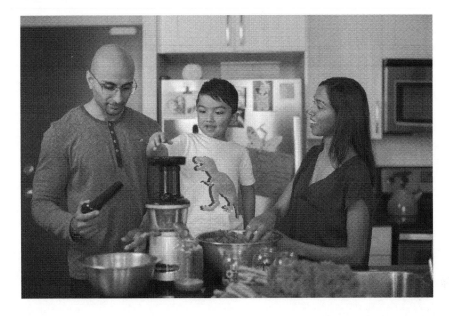

Sachin Patel is a father, husband, philanthropist, practice success coach, speaker, and author. He is on a mission to end the unnecessary suffering that both patients and practitioners are currently experiencing.

His philosophy is that "the doctor of the future is the patient," and he is actively doing whatever it takes to empower people through education, self-care, and remapping of their mindset.

Sachin founded the Living Proof Institute as part of his own personal transformation, and now helps practitioners around the world on how to serve their communities in a deep and meaningful way.

Sachin ensures that practitioners feel appreciated, supported, and empowered in their mission. He provides practical strategies to help his clients attain exceptional outcomes both personally and professionally.

To date, he has delivered hundreds of community workshops and dozens of podcasts and is an advocate for changing the healthcare paradigm. He has devoted his life to the betterment of healthcare for both patients and practitioners.

# Book Sachin Patel to Speak

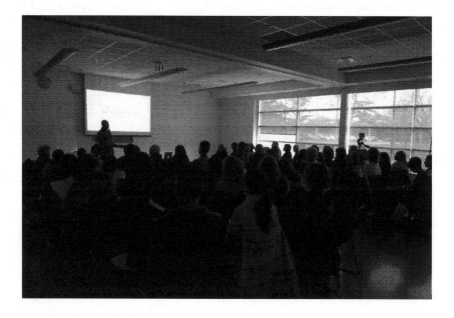

Book Sachin as your keynote, and you're guaranteed to make your event inspirational, motivational, and highly actionable.

Sachin has delivered over 250 live workshops and online events. He has been educating and motivating practitioners and patients from all over the world.

Sachin is a well-recognized leader in the functional medicine space and loves sharing his powerful insights that challenge conventional thinking and force practitioners to take action.

To book Sachin for an event, send an email to info@becomeproof.com.